my big book of healing

Dedication

I would like to dedicate this book to all the people
who have chosen this lifetime to heal.
Your journey is not easy but so worth it.

Remember, it's not about getting to Oz;
it's about the journey on the Yellow Brick Road.

my big book of healing

restore your body, renew your mind, and **heal your soul**

echo bodine

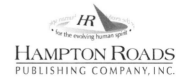

HAMPTON ROADS
PUBLISHING COMPANY, INC.

Cover design by Adrian Morgan
Cover image by iStockphoto

Hampton Roads Publishing Company, Inc.
1125 Stoney Ridge Road
Charlottesville, VA 22902

434-296-2772
fax: 434-296-5096
e-mail: hrpc@hrpub.com
www.hrpub.com

If you are unable to order this book from your local
bookseller, you may order directly from the publisher.
Call 1-800-766-8009, toll-free.
Library of Congress Cataloging-in-Publication Data

Bodine, Echo L.
My big book of healing : restore your body, renew your mind, and heal your
soul / Echo Bodine.
    p. cm.
Rev. ed. of: Passion to heal / Echo L. Bodine.
Summary: "A revised version of Passion to Heal, this is a guide and
workbook to help people overcome physical and mental ailments and
addictions"--Provided by publisher.
ISBN 978-1-57174-588-0 (7 x 9 tp : alk. paper)
1. Mental healing. 2. Mind and body. I. Bodine, Echo L. Passion to heal.
II. Title.
RZ400.B63 2008
615.8'51--dc22

                          2008040731

                 ISBN 978-1-57174-588-0
                 10 9 8 7 6 5 4 3 2 1
          Printed on acid-free paper in the United States

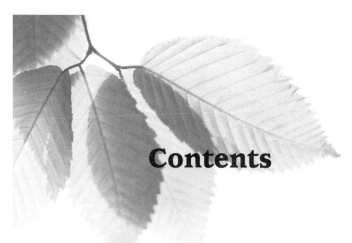

Contents

Acknowledgments   vii
Introduction: From There to Here   ix

Section I: The Inner Work
Chapter 1: Opening to the Healing Journey   3
Chapter 2: Illness: A Wakeup Call   7
Chapter 3: What You Deserve   13
Chapter 4: Nice People Get Sick   17
Chapter 5: Facing the Past   25
Chapter 6: The Inner Child   39

Section II: Obstacles to Healing
Chapter 7: Negative Feelings and Beliefs   51
Chapter 8: Secrets and SECRETS   61
Chapter 9: Addictions and Distractions   69
Chapter 10: Fear and Resentment   81
Chapter 11: Stress and Depression   89

Section III: Gender and Healing
Chapter 12: Women and Their Pain   109
Chapter 13: Men and Their Pain   119

Section IV: Pathways to Healing

Chapter 14: Pregnancy and Parenting   133

Chapter 15: Relationships   145

Chapter 16: Religion   151

Chapter 17: Food and Weight   157

Chapter 18: Grief and Loss   165

Section V: Getting Better

Chapter 19: Finding Solutions   175

Solution 1: Finding a Good Doctor   176

Solution 2: Professional Support   178

Solution 3: Twelve-Step Groups   180

Solution 4: Asking for a Healing   183

Solution 5: t.t.G   185

Solution 6: l.t.G   187

Solution 7: Alternative Healthcare   189

Solution 8: A Positive Attitude   190

Solution 9: Intuition   197

Solution 10: Emotional Release   200

Section VI: Healing as a Way of Life

Chapter 20: Forgiveness   207

Chapter 21: A Better Place   213

Chapter 22: Huckleberry Finn   217

Epilogue   221

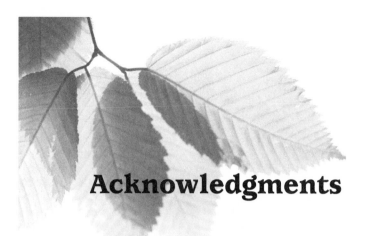

Acknowledgments

I would like to thank the following people for helping me on my journey:

To my dear family, the Bodines. We've been through a lot together, and I'm grateful for all you've given me. I love you.

To my chiropractor and longtime friend, Dr. Marcie New. How can I ever thank you for all of the help you've given to my body, my mind, my emotions, and my soul, as I've moved through my healing process this lifetime?

To Dick Fowler, Mary Teberg, Marilyn Meade-Moore, Rev. Don Clark, Rev. Phil LaPorte, Rev. Ken Williamson, and Lifeworks clinics, for playing a major role in my healing journey.

To my insanely funny (Emperor of the Universe) publisher Greg Brandenburgh for believing in this book and for all your support. You make writing a book a fun adventure.

To Wendy Lazear, an amazing editor with integrity who had the same vision for this book as I've had. Thank you for your beautiful insights and for keeping my voice in the book.

To every one of you very special people, I thank you from the bottom of my heart.

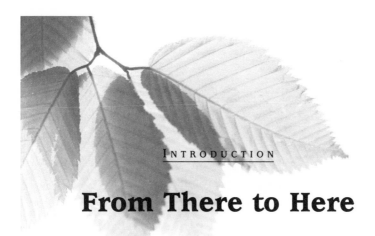

From There to Here

*I*f attempts to find expression fail or are blocked, the
repressed feelings will eventually make your body
sick. It is my belief that most illnesses are caused
by repressed or disowned energies within us.

—Shakti Gawain

The first edition of this book was published in 1993. For
quite a while the Universe had been nudging me to write a book
about the healing process. I kept pretending not to feel those
nudges, remembering how much was involved with writing my
first book, *Hands That Heal* (New World Library). Writing a book
is a lot of work, and I wasn't sure how I was going to say the things
that needed to be said.

I have learned over the years that I always get the higher guidance I need when I ask for it, and this time was no exception. As
the nudges to write this book continued, my course of action was
revealed through a dream that returned for three nights in a row.

The dream was simple: I was standing in front of an Alcoholics Anonymous (AA) meeting, telling my life story to everyone in the group.

Anyone who has ever attended an AA meeting knows that members stand up in front of the group and give testimonials about their lives, telling about how it used to be before AA and how it is now. These stories provide support for everyone who, like the speaker, is in the process of recovering.

After having this dream for the third time, I realized that I was being told that I should share parts of my own healing journey with my readers. I should tell them about growing up in an alcoholic family, being addicted to alcohol and pills, being sexually abused as a child, being an unwed mother, suffering from depression, having poor health during much of my life, and, finally, experiencing my own healing.

In short, I should write a book about my healing journey, as well as the healing journeys of many of my clients.

And so, I begin.

In the Beginning

Let me start by answering two questions that nearly every new client asks me. First, is Echo my real name? Yes, it is. And second, how did I become a healer? The second question is less easy to answer.

When I was seventeen years old and a junior in high school, I went to my first medium for a psychic reading. At the time, I was a typical teenager. I wanted to ask about my future husband and how many children I would have. Would I go to college? If so, which one?

Instead of answering any of these questions, the medium told me that I was born with psychic abilities and the gift of healing. She told me that one day I would be a well-known healer and psychic. I would teach others about their psychic abilities, would write books, and would become known throughout the world. I was stunned.

The medium could "see" other things, too, like the fact that my father was at home that night with a migraine headache. She told me to go home, lay my hands on his head, and ask God to use my hands to heal his headache.

When I got home, I told my dad everything the medium had said and asked him if I could put my hands on his head. He was as nervous and doubtful about this whole thing as I was. The only two healers I'd ever heard about were Jesus and Oral Roberts. You can imagine how tough it was for a shy, seventeen-year-old girl to think of herself as having abilities like theirs!

Nevertheless, my dad agreed to let me place my hands on his head and try to heal him. After twenty seconds my hands started to heat up like little heating pads and trembled a bit. I was scared to death! After about ten minutes, I felt my hands start to cool off. I removed them, and my dad announced that his headache was gone. Gone! No more pain!

That night, I couldn't sleep a wink. I kept wondering, "Why me? What does this mean? Why did God give me this ability?" I felt an overwhelming sense of responsibility. I wondered if news about my healing powers would spread and all the sick people in the world would depend on me to heal them.

As I lay in bed that night I asked God if He would please help me understand. I had always believed in Him, although I didn't know Him very well. Still, I felt confident that the help I was asking Him for would come.

A few weeks later, my psychic abilities began to develop. Every now and then I heard voices—voices that called my name or whispered something only I could hear. I never knew when I was going to hear these voices. They would just come out of nowhere.

One night as I was returning from a friend's home at about 1:30 in the morning, I was about to turn onto Highway 5, the fastest way home. I heard a voice say, "Take Highway 7." The voice seemed so real that I looked in the back seat to see who was there, but nobody was to be seen. As I approached the Highway 5 turnoff, I decided to ignore the voice and take the shorter route, but as I began making the turn I could feel something holding the steering wheel, preventing me from doing so.

I continued toward Highway 7 and then, right across from an all-night gas station, my car had a flat tire. My first reaction was that this was real *Twilight Zone* material. Had I taken Highway 5, which was one of the most sparsely traveled and poorly lit highways in the area, I might have been stranded for a couple of hours.

The voice I'd heard that night and on previous occasions continued to speak to me. I didn't know where it was coming from. But I remembered that the woman who had told me about my gift had also talked to me about spirit guides who would help me along the way. Though I didn't know what this meant, I decided this might be the source of this voice.

For a long time I wandered around afraid, wondering what I was supposed to do with my so-called gifts. In an effort to answer some of the questions I was having, my mom and I took psychic development classes. We even bought a Ouija board and consulted it. We read all of Ruth Montgomery's books. Her *The World Beyond* really helped me to start putting together some of the pieces of the psychic puzzle.

A spiritualist minister in town called my mother one day and told her about a class she was going to teach for people who were psychically gifted. She invited my mom and me to attend. We met every week for nearly a year. I learned a lot about clairvoyance (the gift of seeing visions or images with the third eye—the psychic eye) and clairaudience (hearing messages from the spirits). She taught us about auras (the energy around the body), reincarnation, and karma. The ideas of reincarnation and karma really bothered me. I didn't want to think about life as something I chose. It was easier to blame others or bad luck for the things that seemed to go wrong in my life. I sat on the fence about reincarnation for a long time.

Even as my abilities continued to develop, being "normal" remained very important to me. One of the issues that has always been difficult for me is the expectation that psychics and healers should be kind of weird—dressing oddly, sounding strange, speaking in metaphysical "psychobabble," and living with a black cat in a home that reeks of incense. I didn't want any of that for myself. For a long time, I made a lot of assumptions about spiritual healers, such as:

1. They never get sick because they are so in tune with their bodies.

2. They automatically have a close relationship with God. (It comes with the territory, so to speak.)

3. They have no great challenges in life because they are in some way privileged.

4. They meditate for several hours a day, eat a vegetarian diet, and follow a very rigid exercise program.

5. They are disciplined in their lives.

6. They don't seek material possessions because spirituality and materialism don't mix.

7. They are one step beyond being mere humans.

I'm not sure where I got all these ideas, but they influenced my feelings about myself for many years. I felt like an incredible failure as a healer because I wasn't living up to these standards. I worried that other healers knew something that I didn't.

Again, I asked God for help. Three days later, someone stopped by my office with a flyer announcing that Alberto Aguas, the internationally known healer from Brazil, was coming to Minneapolis to give a healing workshop. I felt compelled to attend.

The three-day workshop was a gift from God. Alberto and I became close friends. He stayed in Minneapolis for a month, and each day we spent some time together. We talked about everything: our lives, our work, our beliefs. I saw the humanness in this world-famous teacher. It was wonderful! Alberto wasn't perfect and didn't pretend to be. He didn't live up to that list of imagined standards for healers any more than I did. He spoke openly of being on his own healing journey.

As time went on, I felt a strong inner peace. I let go of all my silly expectations and accepted my healing abilities. I began to see the truth about people's healing processes, that these were taking so long not because of my shortcomings but because each of us has a process we must go through. The journey of illness and healing is often our best teacher, showing us how to live our lives in a better way. It is rare to discover shortcuts on that path.

Since that time, I have come a long way, both in healing myself and in accepting myself as a healer. Most of the time, I now feel peaceful about my work, my beliefs, and my journey. Most important, I now realize that I have always received whatever I needed along the way to accept my gifts and my humanness.

A Word about What I Do Now

It has been nearly thirty years since I decided to come out of the closet and do psychic work on a full-time basis. One of the toughest challenges has been learning how to live peacefully with my gifts, accepting my psychic abilities while living a normal life. Even now, whenever I fill out an application for a bank account or other services, I flinch when I have to write in my occupation. However, I have found that the more I accept my psychic abilities, the more the world around me accepts them as well.

In the early years, when I was still supporting myself at regular jobs, I did my psychic work in the evenings and on weekends. I was very selective about whom I told of my psychic gifts. I learned early on that many people were uncomfortable about my profession. Some were afraid it might be evil to be psychic. Many people assumed I could read their minds, and they were afraid that being with me would force them to look at their own beliefs and feelings. For all these reasons people would squirm when I told them of my abilities, so for a long time I kept them very private.

Over the years, my method of working has gone through several changes, but some things have remained the same. When I do psychic readings I ask clients to think of questions before they come in for an appointment. When they arrive, I ask them to state their questions. Then I close my eyes, and through breathing and prayer, I go to a calm place within myself. I always ask God to help me bring the client accurate information that will help him the most.

When I first began doing psychic readings, I communicated directly with the client's spirit guides. Guides are loving, compassionate souls who want to help us. They know why we are here and what we are meant to accomplish. Through our thoughts, feelings, and intuition they guide us on our life path. After I contacted these guides, they would give me information about each client.

Later on, I asked God for a spirit guide who would work with me every day, so that I would not have to communicate with a different guide for every person. Shortly after my request, a guide appeared and introduced himself as John Joseph. He explained that he was here to make my life easier.

John was with me for five years, and we had a wonderful relationship. He was a tremendously helpful spirit, and I miss him. He was very loving, funny, and compassionate toward all people. John provided lots of important information for me and my clients, some of which I will share with you in this book.

Over the past forty-two years, the focus of my psychic readings has continually shifted. New guides have come to work with me. Through the information they have provided, I have learned much more about the healing process and the reasons behind our health challenges.

About This Book

This book is very different from my first one, in that the focus is not on my psychic work but on the personal journey that each of us must move through in the process of our own healing. While many books speak of the healing journey and of the need to get down to the emotional roots of our illnesses, there were none that provided a map for this journey. And so it became my goal to provide that map, one that would be a helpful guide for anyone who was looking for a place to begin.

I would like you to think of this as a guidebook for your healing. I highly recommend that you get yourself a book with blank pages that you can use as a journal to keep a permanent record of the exercises at the end of the chapters. Having this record of your journey can be a valuable reference for you as you do this work, one that you will turn to over and over again, reminding you of how far you have come.

Now, let's get on with our healing journey!

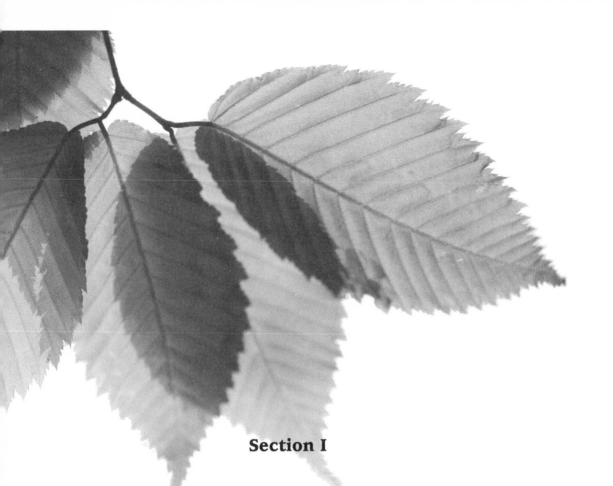

Section I

The Inner Work

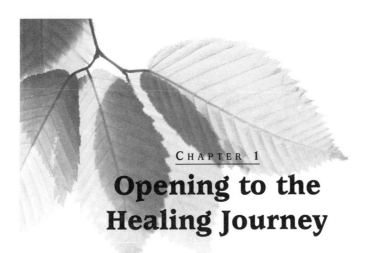

CHAPTER 1

Opening to the Healing Journey

*The experience of illness is a call to a genuinely
religious life. In that sense, it is for many people
one of the best things that ever happened to them.*
—Marianne Williamson

Like most people who have read the Bible, I knew about the miraculous healings performed by Jesus. So when I was told at the age of seventeen that I had the gift of healing, I assumed that people would be instantly and miraculously healed when I laid my hands on them. Yet, as I look back over the past forty-two years of performing spiritual healing, I have seen very few such instant healings. Of course, one explanation for this is that I am not Jesus. But there is another reason too—one that is the focus of this book. Healing is a *process* that involves much more than the physical body. It must occur at many different levels—physical, mental, emotional, and spiritual—for us to be truly healed.

Judy Pearson, one of my former spiritual teachers, introduced me to the idea that most illnesses have emotional roots. She taught me that if we don't address our emotions when we feel them, and if we stuff them instead of expressing them, they won't just go away but will stay inside our bodies and slowly turn into physical problems. Unexpressed feelings and unresolved emotions have no other way to get our attention than for the body to become sick or be in pain.

At first this concept was difficult for me to accept. I was raised with the belief that disease and illness are just a matter of luck. If we are lucky, we don't get sick. Illness randomly strikes us, and there is little or nothing we can do about it except to see a doctor. Worse yet is the belief, held by many, that disease is a form of punishment that comes from God. Judy helped me see that none of these explanations were quite accurate, that we aren't just poor souls who happen to be unlucky and get sick. She was inferring that we each have a role in creating our state of health.

In my practice as a spiritual healer and psychic, I have learned a great deal about people and their health challenges. Above all, I have seen that there are many and varied reasons that we experience such challenges. For most of us, illness can be a tremendous teacher. For some, it is a way to make an exit from life here on Earth.

I am continually reminded of what I have learned from Judy and writers such as Louise Hay and Alice Steadman, whose excellent books have helped me to change my thinking (see *You Can Heal Your Life,* by Louise Hay, and *Who's the Matter with Me,* by Alice Steadman). Their work has helped me to see that I don't have to be a victim who is always asking why life is doing this to me, challenging my health or placing problems in my path; rather, I can start thinking in terms of what I can do to have more choices about my health.

Through my work and the changes I have experienced in my own healing journey, I am continually made aware that most illnesses do have emotional roots and until we look at the unresolved emotions in our lives, our health challenges cannot permanently disappear. We may get temporary relief from a healer, a drug, or even a surgical procedure. Our health challenges may go into remission. The physical pain may stop. But if we don't address the emotions behind an illness, it will remain in our body, only to rear its ugly head at some time in the future.

That's what your healing journey is about: the unresolved emotional pain from the time you were born until today, and what you can do about it. You will learn how to expel all the harmful things you are storing in your body so they can no longer affect your physical health or influence your life in a negative way. Whatever you are storing is keeping you stuck in one way or another. You can go to all the doctors, healers, and health practitioners you want. You can say affirmations until you are blue in the face. You can even pray for miracles. But unless you are willing to feel the unresolved conflicts and pain, explore the negative belief systems, listen to the voice inside, and heal the hurt from your past, *you will stay stuck.* It's all in there. Your whole history is in your body, and it needs to come out to be dealt with consciously.

In the pages ahead, we will look at issues from this lifetime. We will also look at possible solutions, such as what to do if you are sick now, whether it be having therapy, finding a good medical doctor, connecting with an appropriate support group, exploring alternatives in healthcare; or learning more about prayer, meditation, affirmations, forgiveness, and intuition; or finding out how to make new choices in your life that will better support your healing process. We will even explore how to just bring more fun into your life.

As you read this book, and as you do the journal work that it suggests, remind yourself from time to time that this is *your* journey. It is an exciting one. At times it will be painful. But just remember that the pain, which you may experience as you go along, is now sitting in your body. Once you are able to release it, truly release it, you will be free of it forever!

Our illnesses can be our best teachers, guiding us not only to a new freedom from pain but to a better way to live our lives, to a fuller realization of the passion of our true gifts. Allow the process to unfold, and receive whatever it is you need to accept your gifts and yourself. This is perhaps the greatest purpose of the healing journey.

As you embark on this incredible journey, remember that healing does not happen overnight. For most of us, our pain began long ago. When we are able to stay mindful of this and give ourselves all the time we need to do the work, we find the freedom we need to thrive as the children of God that we are.

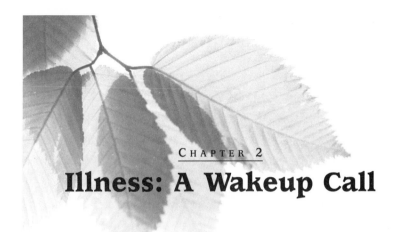

CHAPTER 2

Illness: A Wakeup Call

F*earful as reality is, it is less fearful than evasions of reality.*

—Caitlin Thomas

What would you do if a red light on the dashboard of your car suddenly went on, indicating that something was wrong? Would you wait a few days and hope that the problem resolves itself, in the meantime driving the car? Would you cover up the light with black tape so that you could no longer see it? Or would you take the car to a person who could diagnose the problem and fix it?

When your body has something wrong with it, it has one sure way of letting you know: *pain.* Pain is the body's red warning light. What do you do when the red warning light of pain goes on in your body? Do you wait a few days and hope that the problem will go away? Do you cover it up with pain medication (like putting black tape over the red light on your car)? Or do you pay attention to your body's signals, finding someone who can isolate the cause of the pain and help you get better?

Do you know how many different kinds of pain the body can have? Dull, sharp, throbbing, stabbing, loud, quiet, knifelike (dull or sharp), aching, burning, biting, piercing, severe, stinging, bruising, tender, irritating, inflamed, itching. The body has lots of little voices to tell you when something is wrong. I'm not referring to those slight aches and pains we all have now and then, but to those warning signals that last three days or longer. When the body has a minor pain that lasts more than three days, it needs to be taken seriously. This generally agrees with most medical advice, the three-day period giving your body time to heal itself, after which it may require some additional help. Something is wrong, and your body is trying to get your attention.

Unfortunately, many of us don't take our bodies seriously when they are talking to us. Here are some of the excuses I have heard from clients and friends:

1. I'm too busy to take the time to find out what's wrong.

2. I don't want to be inconvenienced by doctor appointments.

3. I don't want to burden anyone, particularly the doctor.

4. I'm afraid that the doctor won't find anything wrong, and I'll be told it's all in my head.

5. I don't want to hassle with the doctor bills.

6. I don't want to take time off from work.

7. I don't trust doctors.

8. I don't want to know what's wrong.

9. I will go *only* if my insurance company will pay the bills.

10. The pain isn't that bad.

What do you do when your body is sending you warning signals? Is the care you give your body as good as the care you give your car? Have you noticed that you will always find time to fix your car, but often neglect seeing a doctor due to your "busy schedule"? I can just hear some of you saying, "But that's different! I need my car to get around." Yes, but how far are you going to go without a healthy body?

The Importance of Being Still

There are reasons we suffer from pain and illness. Illness is a way for us to get to know ourselves better. It's a tool to change the course of our lives. It's a teacher, a way to find freedom from the past. I strongly believe that pain and illness can be tremendous healers for us when we learn to look at them in a healthy way. And when we learn to *listen* to what our bodies are saying.

The first thing to do when faced with a health challenge is to still your mind. Get away from other people, their stories, their fears, their suggestions for remedies and doctors and healers, their cures and special diets. Get away by yourself so that you can quiet your fears and listen to your body. Get away so that you can listen to your own inner voice. Your illness is trying to speak to you. Be still and listen.

Whenever you are faced with a health challenge, there are solutions. Really, there are! The problem for many of us is that we have internalized the stories of people we knew who had horrible experiences with illness. We think that sharing our pain with others will provide some measure of relief; but it seems that as soon as we tell someone that we need surgery, or that we have cancer, they have a story *to tell us.* This only serves to fuel our fears, and it is very difficult to still our minds when we are full of fear.

When I am doing a healing for a client, I start by clearing all the negative energy that surrounds that person. Much of this negative energy has come from other people who had no intention of sending fear-thoughts. But when you are concerned for your friends or loved ones who are sick, you may be sending them thought-loads of negative energy and fear, despite your loving intentions.

Think about the last time someone told you that she had cancer. When you saw that person again or talked to her on the telephone, what was your first thought? Was it, "How nice to hear from you"? Or was it, "Cancer?" When this happens it's as if you are denying that person's existence, focusing instead on her health challenge.

Soul Learning

I am concerned whenever I encounter the New Age belief that we *create* our illnesses. This type of thinking produces feelings of guilt, shame, and loneliness in the people who are facing health challenges. That's the last thing they need.

I believe we *choose* illness on a soul level as a means of learning. There are no accidents. *Webster's* defines accidents as "unintended events that take place." I believe that everything going on in this world of ours is in Divine Order, so I just can't buy the idea that there are unintended events taking place. Like magnets, we draw whatever happens to us. These "accidents" are full of lessons for our souls, our minds, and our bodies.

Remember that Jesus said, "Love your neighbor as yourself." That means that you come first! Don't sit back and be a victim to whatever physical condition you are facing. The first thing to do when faced with a health challenge is to accept that it is truly happening. Then put on your detective hat and go to work figuring out what might be going on. What is happening in your body? What do you need to do to heal? Treat your body as the most important treasure you have.

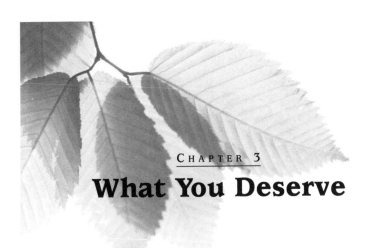

CHAPTER 3

What You Deserve

H*elp me take the blinders off my eyes and see myself clearly.*

—John

Let's look at the word "deserve." I have seen this little seven-letter word mess up more lives! I would love to see it taken out of our vocabulary. *Webster's* defines it as "to be worthy of." But "worthy" is such a heavy word. It gives one a feeling of someone always lurking around us, watching our every move, and then, based on our actions and thoughts, *giving us what we deserve.*

If you're good, you *deserve* something good. If you're bad, you *deserve* something bad. It's that simple . . . and that abusive. "To be worthy of." It seems as if it is always hanging over our heads.

Do I *deserve* happiness?

Have I been good enough to *deserve* that?

Hey, I don't *deserve* that!

I *deserve* to be punished. I'm a sinner.

Oh, he *deserved* everything he got.

If you are physically ill right now, is there a small voice inside your head that says, "I must have done something wrong to deserve this illness"? Who decides what you deserve or don't deserve? Family members? Friends? Co-workers? Your boss? A religious leader? Your significant other? God? Or you?

Whenever we judge whether or not we deserve something, we are usually applying other people's standards. For example, your mother might think that you deserve a new coat, while your father might think that you didn't work hard enough to deserve it. The word "deserve" is about rewards and punishments, guilt and shame. It is about conditional love, which really isn't love at all.

The word "deserve" also diminishes your capacity to heal. Suppose you believe that it was God who decided that you deserved the illness. How good can you be feeling about the chances of your recovery? Why would God be inclined to heal you if He had given you this illness as a form of punishment? Can you see what an impediment the concept of "what you deserve" can be to the healing process? In the next few days, pay attention to how many times you think or say the word "deserve." Pay attention to how many times others use the word, either about themselves or other people. Don't underestimate the effect of this word in your life. It is important to recognize how you feel about this word and the beliefs you have formed in your mind around it.

One reason we cling to our beliefs and feelings around the word "deserve" is that they help us remain in our comfort zone, even if that means blocking our ability to heal. "Secondary gain" is a term psychologists use to describe the payoff people get from clinging to a false belief that reinforces a particular pattern of behavior or negative thought process. The belief allows you to stay in familiar territory, but it threatens your ability to get well.

Here's how it works:

Belief: I don't deserve to have a loving relationship because I cheated on my spouse.

Payoff: I'll never have to commit to a relationship again—which is something I would like to avoid anyway.

Belief: I don't deserve to have nice things in my life because I never take care of them.

Payoff: As long as I hold on to this belief, I will never have to work hard to get nice things.

Belief: I always cheat on my diet, so I don't deserve to be thin.

Payoff: As long as I hold on to this belief, I won't ever have to change my eating habits or take responsibility for my weight problem.

Belief: Because I am a sinner, I don't deserve happiness.

Payoff: As long as I hold on to this belief, I will never really have to open up to life and take risks.

Healing Work

Illness is a way to get to know ourselves. It is a tool to change the course of our lives, a way to find freedom from the past. Pain, illness, and disease are our bodies' way of saying, "Help me to get unstuck. Help me to be free."

In the pages that follow, I will provide exercises to further your healing process. You will be asked to record your observations and impressions in your healing journal. Any notebook will do, although you may want to purchase a special journal that makes you feel connected to the ritual of self-recovery.

To open yourself up to the healing journey, you must first get over any belief that you "deserve" to be sick. Ask your Higher Power to help you let go of the payoffs. Then, as soon as you feel an inner willingness to move forward, which may or may not be right away, ask your Higher Power to heal your negative beliefs. That's right. Simply *ask* that they be healed. Sound too easy? Do you have a difficult time believing that you deserve it to be that simple? Give that up, too! Be willing to move forward *now*.

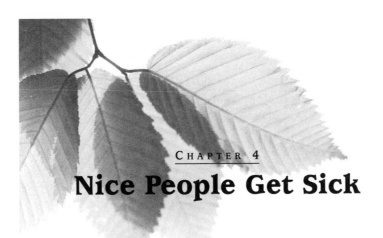

CHAPTER 4

Nice People Get Sick

*I*f *you go up to any head nurse on a ward and point to two women who came in with lumps in their breasts and one is a pain in the neck and driving everyone crazy and another is this wonderful, gentle, little lady who is doing everything that everybody wants, and you ask which one has cancer, the nurse is going to say the sweet, gentle one. The nice people always get cancer. But, you see, the definition of nice is the people who won't express themselves, who won't express rage and anger and who internalize it and then get depressed and then get sick.*

—Bernie Siegel, MD

How many times have you heard people ask, "Why do nice people get cancer?" Or they say, "Cancer always happens to such nice people!" The quote above, from a best-selling author and Yale surgeon, explains why. Nice people are frequently people who have trouble expressing themselves, and the evidence suggests that there is a strong link between illness and the inability to express what's inside.

Does this mean that everyone who is nice is going to get cancer? Of course not. But the truth is that there does seem to be a strong link between illness and not being able to express one's self.

Several years ago, Michael, a college professor, came to me seeking relief from his pain. He had recently suffered two heart attacks and a stroke that left him partially paralyzed on his left side. The first thing he said to me after introducing himself was that he was a Christian and that he had always tried to help people as much as he could. He seemed very gentle and loving. He was also an intelligent man who was sincere about his desire to heal himself. While I was channeling the healing to him, John, my spirit guide, said to me, "Yes, he has been a 'Christian' to everyone else, but has forgotten about himself."

Christine, a high school teacher, came to me for a healing on her neck. It had suddenly become stiff, preventing her from being able to move her head from side to side. When I placed my hands on her neck, I saw the image of a man sitting there, inside of her. She appeared to have become "fused" with this man, always anticipating his wants and needs, always focused on him. She'd forgotten about herself. He consumed her thoughts, her time, her life.

I saw another image, too, this one of Christine herself, yelling, "Hey, what about me?" I could see that there was a tremendous internal conflict between Christine and this man. Should she be true to herself or to him? If she didn't make him the center of her life, would he leave her? The pain in her body was saying, "He is a total pain in the neck, get him out of here." I knew that she needed to break this cycle and that she would probably not be able to do this on her own. Regrettably, I saw her only once. But if she is like many other clients I have seen with similar patterns in their relationships, she sought out and received the kind of help she needed.

Heal Thyself

Does it sound as if I am suggesting that we shouldn't be nice, loving, or nurturing? If so, that is certainly not my intent. The problem comes when we are nice to other people at our own expense. Healthy people take responsibility for themselves, making certain their own needs are met. Then they take the extra energy they get from taking care of themselves and use it to be there for others. "Nice" people use up all of their energy taking care of others and end up with nothing left for themselves. Usually what follows is illness, which is one of the only ways "nice" people have of feeling cared for. The greatest loss "nice" people suffer is their loss of self.

I used to be a "nice" person, paying more attention to the wants and needs of others than to myself. When asked about my feelings or thoughts on a particular subject, my immediate reaction was always confusion. I had no idea what to think or feel on my own. For example, when my boyfriend asked me what I wanted to do on Saturday night, I would first try to figure out what it was *he* wanted to do and then give him the answer I thought would make him happy. I placed his needs before my own, sacrificing my own health in the process.

"Nice" people act in the name of charity and kindness, but their deeper motivation stems from a poor self-image or lack of self-worth. They don't think they have a right to put themselves first or to have their own opinions. Moreover, it is very difficult for them to imagine that anyone else would care what they believed.

If you recognize yourself as a "nice" person, it is essential to your health to break this pattern. Low self-esteem, self-destructiveness, and self-hatred all have their roots in self-denial. Instead, you need to fight, and fight hard, for yourself. I really do believe that the destructive pattern of caretaking, people-pleasing, and martyrdom—the way many of us have of being the rescuer to everyone else but ourselves—is at the root of a lot of illnesses.

Remember what Jesus said: "Love thy neighbor as thyself." The bottom line is that we each deserve and need love and caring. Someone once said that the most valuable thing we have to give is ourselves. But what if there is no self to give? Then, the gift we try to pass along to others is going to be of no use to anyone. In a very real way, our primary responsibility is to put ourselves first.

Getting beyond "Nice"

Learning to say no is the first step toward getting and staying healthy. It may be difficult at first, just as it was difficult learning to walk. But gradually, you will see that learning to say no is a self-strengthening step that leaves you with no one else's life to maintain but your own. Once you let go of the responsibility for other people's lives, you will no longer be silently resentful, envious, angry, or miserable, and you already know what happens to all that negativity sitting inside of your body. Eventually, it erupts into pain or illness.

CHARACTERISTICS OF "NICE" PEOPLE

You are "nice" if you:

- are unable to distinguish your own thoughts and feelings from those of others (you think for and feel responsible for other people)
- seek the approval and attention of others in order to feel good
- feel anxious or guilty when others "have a problem"
- do things to please others even when you don't want to
- do not know what you want or need
- rely on others to define your wants or needs
- believe that others know what is best for you better than you do
- throw temper tantrums or collapse when things don't work out the way you expect them to
- focus all your energy on other people and on their happiness
- try to prove to others that you are good enough to be loved
- are unable to believe you can take care of yourself
- believe that everyone else is trustworthy. You idealize others and are disappointed when they don't live up to your expectations
- whine or pout to get what you want
- feel unappreciated and unseen by others
- blame yourself when things go wrong
- think you are not good enough
- fear rejection by others
- live your life as if you are a victim of circumstances
- feel afraid of making mistakes
- wish others would like or love you more
- try not to make demands on others
- are afraid to express your true feelings for fear that people will reject you

- let others hurt you without trying to protect yourself

- are unable to trust yourself and your own decisions

- find it hard to be alone with yourself

- pretend that bad things aren't happening to you, even when they are

- keep busy so you don't have to think about things

- don't need anything from anyone

- experience people and life as black and white—either all good or all bad

- lie to protect and cover up for people you love

- feel very scared, hurt, and angry but try not to let it show

- find it difficult to be close to others

- find it difficult to have fun and to be spontaneous

- feel anxious most of the time and don't know why

- feel compelled to work, eat, drink, or have sex even when you don't seem to get much enjoyment from the activity

- worry that other people will leave you

- feel trapped in relationships

- feel you have to coerce, manipulate, beg, or bribe others to get what you want

- cry to get what you want

- feel controlled by the feelings of others

- are afraid of your own anger

- feel helpless and powerless to change yourself or your situation

- think someone else needs to change in order for you to feel better

Journal Work

In your journal, make any notes you wish about this issue and how it affects you. Think about specific relationships in your life: Are there people whom you are always trying to please or whose needs you are always putting before your own? Are there people whose "niceness" makes you uncomfortable? Do you ever feel guilty about these people? If you feel that there are many of these types of relationships in your life, make some notes about each of them, using the above list as a guide.

Remember, being "nice" is no excuse for neglecting your health and well-being. To God, you are just as deserving as the next guy. Start believing it.

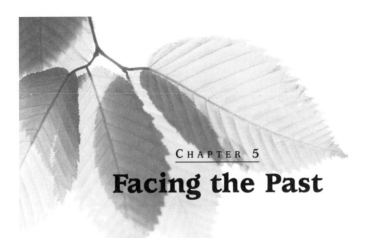

CHAPTER 5

Facing the Past

A journey of a thousand miles must begin with a
single step.

—Lao-tzu

Where do we begin in the healing process? At the beginning! Some therapists believe that the past is neither important
nor relevant in a person's healing process. If you are a person
who doesn't want to go back to your painful past, the chances
are that you will be drawn to such a therapist. You may learn
new "coping skills," how to "control" your emotions, and how
to say no to the past. But this will keep you going around in circles, staying stuck right where you are. Every person I've ever
known who has gone this route, whether friend or client, has
remained stuck.

The healing process that I am recommending in this book
does not involve dredging up the past, rehashing it over and over,
and then staying there. Instead, I'm talking about going back,
honestly looking at your memories, feelings, and emotional pain,

then discussing what you've learned with a professional or close friend who can help you let go of the pain that may be stuck in your body.

Paul, a young man of about thirty-seven, came to me for a healing involving his chronic back pain. His doctors couldn't find anything wrong, yet they had prescribed many different pain killers. Paul wanted a different solution. His back pain was causing problems in his marriage. He was irritable most of the time, and he had become very critical of his wife and everything she did. He had been forced to quit his job as a store manager because of his constant pain and because he was always high on medication.

When I placed my hands on his back, it felt "full." My impression was that it was swollen with emotions. I looked inside psychically and saw an older man who was filled with rage and was yelling and hitting a young boy. I saw terror in the boy's eyes, and I saw his feelings of powerlessness and hatred for the older man.

I asked Paul if his father had beaten him, and he said yes. Had his father been an alcoholic? Yes, again. I told him that all of his anger, resentments, fear, and the trauma he suffered growing up in that environment were in his back. I got a very strong sense that he needed more help than I was able to give him with the laying-on-of-hands healing.

I asked him if he had ever talked to a therapist or pastor about his childhood. He said that he had not, replying that "what's in the past stays in the past." Paul truly believed, as so many of us do, that because our childhoods are out of sight, they are out of mind (and body). But as I have seen time after time, that simply is not true.

Going Back

Many people think that going back to their past and dredging up all the pain isn't going to do any good. Unfortunately, these are usually the people who need to do it the most!

Yes, it's hard. It's painful. I would rather have done a thousand other things than to go back and look at what it was I was trying so hard to forget. I spent years dodging the pain I stuffed inside. I distracted myself as much as possible from experiencing the feelings of the past and present. I believe this is why I have suffered so many health problems since childhood.

This chapter is about your childhood. My childhood. Your beginning. My beginning. This is where many physical problems, if you have them, probably got started . . . a long time ago. The hurt, the pain, the abuse, the injustices we suffered as children, all got stored in our bodies if we were unable to let the feelings out at the time. Many of us were not taught to express our feelings because our parents and grandparents didn't know how to express theirs. We were taught to keep our mouths shut. "Kids are to be seen and not heard." "Don't whine." "Don't cry." "Don't talk back (because your opinion doesn't count)." "Be sweet." "Be cute." "Be the perfect child." "Always smile, even when you are disappointed." "If your feelings get hurt, swallow them." "Be a big boy." "Be a big girl."

In many cases, food or other rewards were used to soothe the feelings we were discouraged from expressing. Those of us who grew up in dysfunctional families—which is just about everyone, as it turns out—never knew that we mattered or that we were lovable and acceptable. We didn't feel a sense of safety or that we could trust our parents or caregivers to be there for us. The world appeared to be a scary, unpredictable, untrustworthy, and inconsistent place.

Every child needs to be loved unconditionally. When we don't get the love, attention, and affection we need while we are growing up, we may have difficulty with our relationships later in life. On my own healing journey, I came to see how my dysfunctional childhood had greatly affected my later life. I came to understand that much of the time I was reacting not from the place of being a full-grown adult but out of the neediness, confusion, trauma, wants, and fears of a child.

Family Secrets

It is the curse of the child from a dysfunctional background to feel protective of the family and its secrets. Being the firstborn in our family, I found this to be particularly true. Our family had a great sense of pride in being able to take care of each other and not need anyone else. Even as I write this chapter, the old curse of wanting to protect the family surfaces. I find it difficult to write these words.

There was emotional, physical, and sexual abuse in my dysfunctional family system. It has been difficult for me over the years to be open with myself or others about how insane our family life became at times. I always minimized it. I always wanted to protect myself from being abandoned, so I never rocked the boat. But all my efforts to protect what little I had only prolonged my poor health, my poor relationships, my low self-worth, and the negative attitudes and feelings I had developed about myself.

When I entered therapy, it became necessary for me to stop protecting the family pain and start paying more attention to my own feelings. I had to give up my misplaced sense of loyalty and protectiveness toward the family in order to heal.

If you are anything like me, you may not even know about the abuse you suffered as a child. Some of us do such a good job of hiding the truth from others that we end up hiding it from ourselves. To help me discover what might have happened to me, my therapist gave me a list of abusive actions. These included actions that might have been done to me by others as well as abusive actions I might have taken against myself.

Pay attention to your reactions as you read over the list. Do you find yourself minimizing any of them, perhaps making excuses for those who abused you or telling yourself that their abuse didn't really hurt you? These tendencies to downplay what occurred are the natural reactions of anyone who has suffered such treatment. But remember, abuse is abuse. Nothing on this list is good for us. Be honest with yourself as you read over this list, reminding yourself that if you are attempting to make light of anything you read here, the chances are very good that you are reacting to a deep pain you suffered in the past.

PHYSICAL ABUSE

Slapping; spanking; shaking; scratching; squeezing; beating with board, stick, belt, kitchen utensil, yardstick, electrical cord, shovel, or hose.

Throwing, pushing, shoving, slamming against walls or objects; burning, scalding, freezing; forcing of food or water, starving; having to watch others being physically abused; overworked.

SEXUAL ABUSE

Fondling, touching, innuendoes, jokes, comments, looking, being exposed to masturbation, mutual masturbation, oral sex, anal sex, intercourse, penetration with fingers or objects, stripping and sexual punishments, pornography—either taking pictures of you or forcing you to look at such pictures. Forcing children into sexual acts with each other, forced sexual activity involving animals, watching others have sex or be abused, sexual "games," sexual torture (such as burning), etc.

VERBAL ABUSE

Excessive guilting, blaming, shaming, name-calling, putting-down, comparing, teasing, making fun of, laughing at, belittling, nagging, haranguing, screaming, verbally assaulting.

PHYSICAL NEGLECT

Lack of food, clothes, shelter; leaving the child alone; leaving a child who is too young in charge of others; failure to provide medical care; allowing or encouraging the use of drugs or alcohol; failure to protect a child from abuse from others.

EMOTIONAL ABUSE

Projection and transfer of blame (being punished for the parent's own shortcomings); alterations of the child's reality (an adult telling a child that an experience he had didn't really occur— "Mama didn't beat you—you made that up"). Overprotecting, smothering, excusing, blaming others for child's problems; fostering and encouraging low self-esteem; conditional love ("Mommy won't love you anymore if you misbehave"). Double messages (one parent telling you one thing, the other telling you just the opposite). Refusing to talk about abuse at all.

It is estimated that one out of every eight Americans is a child of an alcoholic. That means there are approximately 28 million wounded, adult children out there! And that only includes the children of alcoholic parents. What about the rest? What about the children of sex addicts? Drug addicts? Codependents? Gamblers? Overeaters? Religious fanatics? And what about the children of parents who are emotionally unstable but don't have obvious addictions? The numbers are staggering. Where does one begin the healing process? At the beginning . . . with the first step.

In their book *The Secrets of Dysfunctional Families,* John and Linda Friel provide the following list of roles in a dysfunctional family system.

THE DO-ER

The Do-er is always *doing,* making certain the daily needs of the family are being met; making sure the children are fed, bathed, and dressed; paying the bills; ironing the clothes; doing the shopping; taking the kids to Little League or music lessons. But because the family is dysfunctional, all this consumes the Do-er's time and energy, leaving her little or no time for anything else. So the Do-er feels tired and lonely. She may feel that others take advantage of her, and as a result may feel emotionally neglected and empty. Such a person gets a lot of satisfaction out of being so accomplished, being able to accomplish so much, and other members of the family encourage the Do-er, either directly or indirectly. Meanwhile, the Do-er's own guilt and overdeveloped sense of responsibility keeps her *doing, doing, doing.*

THE ENABLER/HELPER/LOVER

The Enabler/Helper/Lover nurtures other family members and provides them with a sense of belonging. Often this person is also the Doer, but not always. The goal of the Enabler/Helper/Lover is to keep everyone together, preserving the family unit at any cost, even if it means suffering physical violence or even death. The Enabler/Helper/Lover is always trying to avoid conflict in the family, spending a lot of time and energy trying to smooth ruffled feathers. People who take on this role are often motivated by fear of abandonment and fear that other family members cannot stand on their own two feet.

THE LOST CHILD/LONER

The Lost Child/Loner is the one who stays to herself a lot. She may stay in her room or spend time out of doors, playing in the woods by herself. This person is actually making an effort to act out a need for separateness and autonomy that most other members of the dysfunctional family feel. But while she may spend a lot of time alone, it is not a healthy aloneness because most of her time is spent trying to escape both the family and the feelings she has around it. This person usually feels a deep sense of loneliness that she carries into adulthood—or until her early feelings are resolved.

THE HERO

The Hero provides the family with self-esteem. He may go off to law school and become a famous attorney, but in his heart he may secretly feel awful because his sister is in a mental hospital and his younger brother has died of alcoholism. Heroically, he carries the family banner for all the world to see, making the family proud. But all of this is accomplished at a terrible price in terms of his own well-being, since he feels burdened by the weight of his impossible task.

THE MASCOT

The Mascot is often a younger child. She provides comic relief for the family. The Mascot uses humor to give the family a sense of playfulness, silliness, fun, and a kind of distorted joy. The cost to the Mascot is that her true feelings of isolation and pain never get expressed. Until she gets into recovery or another program, she remains an emotional cripple.

THE SCAPEGOAT

The Scapegoat is the person who acts out all the family's dysfunction, taking the blame for the rest of them. He may be the black sheep of the family, using drugs, stealing, getting into fights, or acting out sexually. All of this "bad behavior" from this one person then allows the other family members to say, "If little brother would just straighten himself up, we'd be a healthy family." The cost to the Scapegoat is that he may spend a lifetime caught up in negative behavior and self-abuse.

DAD'S LITTLE PRINCESS/MOM'S LITTLE MAN

This child is seduced, early on, by a parent who is too afraid or dysfunctional to get her needs met by other adults. Adored as long as we acted out the parent's model of the ideal, loving, talented child, we are never appreciated for who we really are, nor are our own childhood needs respected. Those of us who fell into this role as children usually ended up getting physically or emotionally abused by other adults in later life because our boundaries and our needs were not respected when we were little.

THE SAINT/PRIEST/NUN/RABBI

This child takes on the family's religious or spiritual needs and often becomes a priest, nun, rabbi, or monk. One of the conditions that may go along with this role is to live a life of denial, particularly abstinence from sex. The family may do nothing obvious to mold the person into this role, though it is implied, subtly reinforced, and silently encouraged. This child nevertheless grows up believing that he will win a sense of self-worth only if he takes on the spiritual/religious needs of the family.

Do you identify with any of these roles? In your journal you might want to make some notes about which ones you identify with and why. It is also worth noting here that you might identify with a combination of these roles, being a Do-er, a Hero, and a Saint, all in one. Or you might vacillate between one role and another, being a Lost Child/Loner in some circumstances, a Scapegoat in others. In any case, take a close look at all of these characteristics and see how they relate to you.

Finishing Up

Many changes will take place during your healing journey. There will be times when doing the inner work will be emotionally painful. You will experience a lot of feelings. You will be getting to know yourself in a different way. You will be releasing some old patterns and beliefs. Be conscious of the fact that what you feel is the pain you are bringing to the surface, and that has been stored in your body for years and years. In letting it out, you are doing a wonderful cleansing of your body and soul.

Be patient. Give yourself plenty of breaks. When I was writing this book, I had to completely walk away and do something light. Yes, we want to get to the stored pain in order to free ourselves of it. But we didn't take on that pain overnight—and we won't get rid of it overnight, either!

When you are done with the journal exercises at the end of each section, I strongly recommend that you do something physical to work the feelings out of your body. Or just take yourself out and do something fun. (See chapter 22 for suggestions.)

You may also wish to share your feelings with a friend or confidant whom you think you can trust or consult a good therapist (more on this in chapter 19). Don't think that you have to do it alone. Incorporate the exercises in this book into any additional therapy or course of healing you decide to do.

Above all, be as loving as you can to yourself. Be gentle and understanding. You're doing a great job. Keep going!

Journal Work

Exercise 1

A Picture of Your Past

Use your journal to begin making notes about your childhood. If you are having trouble remembering your childhood, go through some family photo albums. Ask your grandparents or old family friends if they remember any stories about you as a child. Talk to friends with whom you grew up. If you have toys or other mementos from your childhood, these can also help stimulate memories of that time.

Some of the questions you might ask yourself are: What messages did you receive as a child about expressing your feelings? Were you encouraged to speak your mind or to keep quiet? What did you do when you felt fear, anger, sadness, or discouragement, or when your feelings were hurt? Whenever you did express your feelings, did anyone listen? Did they act as if they cared about what you were feeling?

Look at the ways you were taught to express, or not express, positive feelings as well as the so-called negative ones. I'm talking about positive emotions such as joy, excitement, love, and happiness. Were your needs and wants respected? Did you feel people listened to you?

Note in your journal how it feels to you now as you think back and feel your childhood memories. What sticks out as the most painful memory or memories? Did your parents want a boy, and you turned out to be a girl—or vice versa? Was the fact that you turned out to be the gender you are a disappointment to them?

If you were raised by a single parent, did you in any way feel you were expected to be a surrogate spouse? Were you allowed to be a child, or did you feel you had to be mature and responsible no matter what your age? If you had brothers and sisters, were you expected to be responsible for them?

Was there physical abuse in the family? Sexual abuse? Was there a sense in your family that you didn't need any outsiders, that all you needed was each other?

Write it all down. All of it! The resentments. The sadness. The anger. Take your time—please don't think you have to do the whole thing in one sitting. What you discover here is important to your health—mentally, emotionally, and physically. If you need to spread this work out over several days or even a few weeks, that's okay.

Exercise 2

Childhood Health History

Record in your journal any health problems you had as a child, other than the usual childhood diseases. Do you still suffer from any of them? It can be helpful to ask one of your parents if they remember any specific events that occurred around the same time that you had an illness. Illnesses such as asthma, digestive problems, and mood swings can often have strong links with early events in our lives. Sometimes these show up quite dramatically when I begin working with a client.

You might find it helpful to divide a page in your journal into two columns. Label the first column "Childhood Illnesses" and the second one "Emotional Events." As you remember each illness, list any emotional events that might have been associated with that illness, particularly those that occurred just prior to any symptoms appearing for the first time.

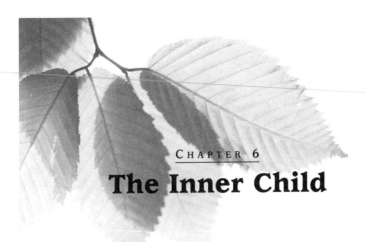

CHAPTER 6

The Inner Child

Each of us has a child within, a part of us that is sensitive, vulnerable, playful, sweet, innocent, giggly, squirmy, creative, lovable, curious, smiling, and filled with wonder. Even if you don't allow yourself to express this part, your inner child is still there—wanting and needing attention, recognition, acceptance, love, nurturance, and joy.

How do you experience joy? Do you allow yourself to get excited? Feel silly? Laugh? Do you ever take your shoes off and wiggle your toes in the water? Blow bubbles with bubble gum? Buy yourself balloons? Swing on a swing? Slide down a slide? Run through the sprinkler? Roast marshmallows on a stick over the fire? Go to an amusement park and allow yourself to see through your inner child's wondering eyes? When was the last time you flew kites or a balsawood airplane? Or colored a picture with crayons? It doesn't matter what age you are today. The child within is still there. It needs to be recognized in order for you to feel whole and complete.

Many of us didn't get our needs met as children. We were never acknowledged for who we were. Rather, we were told who we were supposed to be. Some of us were told not to be playful, imaginative, creative, curious, giggly, or wondering. Others lost their innocence through abuse or neglect. When our childhood needs for love, nurturing, and acceptance aren't met, we grow up feeling as if there is something wrong with us. We feel lopsided. Empty. Full of holes, like Swiss cheese.

Developing a relationship with your inner child is very important for your healing process. In doing so, you will learn about yourself and will feel much more complete and whole. Whether you acknowledge your inner child or not, the fact remains that it continues to exist, influencing how you feel and what you do in your everyday life.

John Bradshaw, author of the best-selling books *Bradshaw On: The Family* and *Healing the Shame That Binds You,* stated in *New Realities* magazine (July/August 1990): "The neglected wounded inner child is the major source of human misery," and that this is "the major cause of addictions and addictive behavior. When our inner child is wounded, we feel empty and depressed. Life has a sense of unreality about it; we are there, but we are not in it. This emptiness leads to loneliness. Because we are never who we really are, we are never truly present."

If your inner child was wounded, not getting love or positive recognition, there's a very good chance that this same inner child is still very needy today. This neediness will affect your relationships with nearly everyone around you. Maybe the only time you were ever recognized as a child was when you were playing a trick on someone or hurting someone in a kidding way. Maybe you were noticed by getting yelled at or even punished, but at least you were noticed! As an adult, you may still be getting attention in similar ways. The problem is that people can't trust you. They're always on their guard because your inner child doesn't know how to ask for attention or affection in ways that are mutually satisfying.

Perhaps as a child, you were never allowed to talk about your feelings. Twenty-five years later, your boss calls you into her office to tell you about a mistake you made. Your inner child takes over. "Nobody appreciates me! Everyone hates me," it cries. You feel so full of rage that you could easily do something self-destructive— quit your job, or get drunk, or get into your car and drive it off the road. These are the kinds of self-abusive acts that will continue to occur until you are able to give your inner child the love and attention it needs.

You may have been sexually abused as a child and kept it all inside, not knowing how to talk about it or not having anyone you could trust to share what you were feeling. This made you feel powerless and confused. As an adult, you may act out these feelings by being very aggressive or promiscuous, desperately trying to feel sexually powerful. The inner child, in an effort to get back at the perpetrator for being made to feel so full of shame, now uses its sexuality to hurt everyone possible.

Maybe as you were growing up you felt no sense of protection from those around you. The only way you felt safe was by surrounding yourself with layers and layers of protection. You developed a weight problem. And now, no matter how many diets you try or how much weight you lose, that weight comes right back. It will continue to do so until your inner child can feel safe.

Perhaps when you were small, no one listened to you. So you learned to make your stories more interesting by lying or exaggerating. As an adult, you are still lying and exaggerating your stories in order to get people to listen to you. The problem is that eventually people will catch onto your lies and won't listen to you anyway!

Maybe when you were young, you only received physical affection when you were sick. That same effort to get affection can carry over into adulthood, this time becoming the source of illnesses that are life-threatening.

Are you wondering how to recognize the cries of your own inner child? My therapist gave me an excellent suggestion for doing this. Whenever you are in a situation that has brought up feelings such as fear, anger, rage, sadness, confusion, despair, hopelessness, or terror, ask yourself how old you feel. That's right! How old do you feel at the time you are experiencing these emotions? You may feel three, six, or twelve years old, or you may even feel as if you are an infant who can't speak and is totally dependent on others. This is very helpful in knowing if you're reacting from the child's or the adult's feelings.

In my own effort to understand more about how to feel, know, and embrace the inner child, I discovered Lucia Capacchione's book, *Recovery of Your Inner Child,* which helped me learn to access my inner child in a wonderfully simple way. For those of you who are intellectual, these exercises may be difficult, but I ask you to open your mind to these ideas.

Capacchione suggests having a dialogue with your inner child. First take yourself somewhere that children like to go and begin the dialogue by letting the child within draw a picture, similar to the ones you may have drawn in kindergarten. After your inner child has drawn a picture, start dialoguing by writing a question to it with your dominant hand. For instance, ask your inner child, "How are you today?" Let the child respond by writing with your nondominant hand. Here is an example of what my inner child wrote:

I am fine   I am afraid

I am happy   I am mad

I am sad   I don't know

Capacchione warns that we all have within us a critical parent who may try to sabotage this experience. Your critical or shaming parent may say things like:

"Hurry up, you're too slow!"

"Your penmanship is messy."

"That's a stupid thing to say."

"You're dumb."

"Your opinion is stupid."

"I have more important things to do than listen to you."

"I'm in a hurry, let's go."

"You're just a child, what do you know?"

Listen to your inner parent with the realization that the way it parents your inner child reveals something to you about how you were parented as a child. Without feeling that you have to act on what this inner parent is saying, simply take note of what it is saying. Go beyond this critical voice by paying attention to your inner child's own needs for affection and recognition; right now, these are more important than meeting the needs of the inner parent.

Remember that it's important to allow the child to come out at its own pace. When we meet a small child, we are gentle in our conversation with him. We don't push the child or force him to have a relationship with us. By the tone of our voice and mannerisms, we are trying to convey that he is cared for and safe. We need to treat our own inner child in the same way.

Tell your inner child that you recognize that it may not have felt protected but that now, as an adult, you will provide that protection. You will create a safe environment. The inner child needs to feel safe in order to talk with you about its feelings. It is up to you, as the adult, to give that child the safety, the protection, the reassurance, the attention, the acknowledgment that it (you) did not get earlier. Your inner child deserves to have all of these!

If you are wondering how you are going to do this, think about any small children you may know right now. If any of these children came to you needing to feel safe, loved, and acknowledged, how would you provide that support? You are going to have to learn how to do the same for yourself.

Inner-Child Play

I would like to suggest that you buy some big crayons or markers that will help you and your inner child dialogue in your journal. Once I began dialoguing with my inner child, we went on for pages and pages!

If you have children of your own, don't use their tablets or crayons. Get a set for your own inner child! I took myself to a park that I went to as a child. I had no specific memories, but I felt childlike sitting in a park on a blanket. I immediately began drawing trees. The feeling I had was familiar, even though I hadn't experienced it for a long time. It was an excited feeling. My mind filled with ideas for my picture: the sun, the sky, a house. My imagination overtook my intellect. I switched crayons two or three times. It was fun.

Of course, my critical parent was there saying, "Oh, this is ridiculous. I should be home cleaning the house or doing laundry." I jotted down these critical comments on a separate piece of paper (with my dominant hand to save time) and continued on with my picture.

Suddenly, I became bored with my picture and wanted to do something else. I grabbed a pen with my dominant hand and wrote out a question to my inner child.

Adult: Are you really there?
My nondominant hand grabbed a blue crayon and said, Yes!
Adult: How are you today?
Inner Child: Happy.
Adult: Why are you happy?
Inner Child: Because we're at the park.
Adult: How old are you?
Inner Child: Four.

I asked my inner child simple questions about its feelings on different topics. Some of its replies were a single word. Others were more elaborate. Capacchione suggests asking the inner child what it would like to be called. Mine came up with "Little Echo," a name my dad still calls me at times today.

When you are ready to finish a dialogue with your inner child, tell it that you want to become more aware of it throughout your daily life. Ask for a code, a way to let you (the adult) know that it wants or needs to talk with you. Little children love codes, remember? Mine said it would think of the color red. This has worked very well. Whenever I hear or sense an inner nudging of red, red, red, I grab my tablet and ask my inner child, "What's up?" It always has something to say.

As you come to the end of this chapter and read the journal exercises I've included there, you may think at first that they are pretty dumb! But as silly as these exercises may seem, they are wonderfully freeing.

By doing these exercises, you will meet a very important person in your life: your own inner child from your past, the child that still exists within you. Allow yourself to feel excited about this wonderful new relationship. This child is brimming over with love for your adult self.

Love this inner child. You're the adult now. You can give your inner child everything it ever wanted or needed—love, recognition, acceptance, someone to listen to it. Acknowledging this inner child, nurturing this relationship, can fill up those empty spaces inside. You will feel more complete. The unmet needs of your inner child will no longer control your life. You will feel in control of yourself and will be able to choose the way you want to live. You won't continually embarrass yourself with actions that you don't understand.

If you have not previously looked at the wounds of your inner child, it may not be very happy when you first make contact. Your inner child may feel very hurt, neglected, mistrustful, sad, alone, ashamed, or unwanted. Your child may want to tell you how lonely it has been or how hard it was when you were little. Allow the child to say anything that it needs or wants to say. Give it all the time and space it needs.

This inner child is not separate from you. This child is an important part of you!

Journal Work

As you start this work with your inner child, you may want to consider keeping a box of paper, crayons, and pencils set aside for your inner-child work. This would be in addition to the journal you will be keeping. Let your inner child help you choose these materials, making certain there is enough so that it can fill up many pages with drawings or dialogue.

Think about the way small children draw and write. With your nondominant hand you will do the same, and if you only have your journal available for this you may feel somewhat reluctant to fill as many pages as you might want to do.

Exercise 1

Draw a Picture

On a separate sheet of paper, or in your journal, ask your inner child to draw a picture. Use your nondominant hand to express your inner child. Let the child pick out whatever color crayon it wants.

If your inner child is angry, it may draw an unhappy or angry picture, a mean or scary picture. Assure your inner child that it is okay to express itself in any way it chooses.

Exercise 2

Dialogue with Your Inner Child

After you are done drawing a picture, ask your inner child any questions that you would like. You can write these questions out with your dominant hand. Then turn the pen or crayon over to your nondominant hand so that your inner child can write the answers.

Exercise 3

What Is Your Inner Child's Name?

Ask your inner child what it would like to be called. The name your inner child comes up with may surprise you, or it may be a name you were called when you were a child.

With your nondominant hand, have your inner child record this name in your journal.

Exercise 4

Record Messages from Your Critical Parent

Remember to watch for your critical parent. When you hear or feel its critical messages, make a mental note of them. Then, using your dominant hand, record them in your journal.

Exercise 5

Your Inner Child's Secret Code

With your dominant hand, ask your inner child for a code that will let you know when it wants to communicate with you. Then let your inner child choose a pen, pencil, or crayon to record its code in your journal.

As you come to the end of a session with your inner child, thank it for its picture and for sharing its feelings. Assure the child that you will continue to listen to it and that its opinion is very important to you. End your conversation in whatever way seems most comfortable to you.

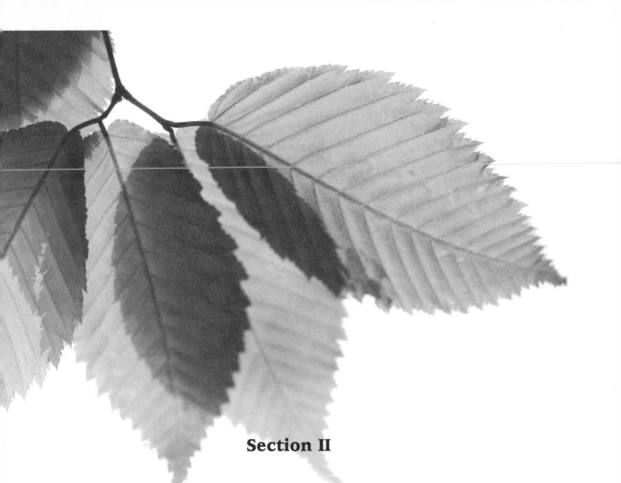

Section II

Obstacles to Healing

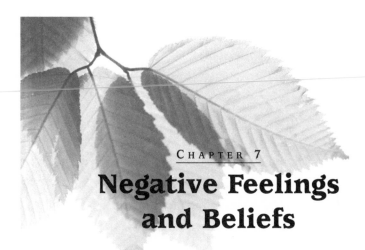

CHAPTER 7

Negative Feelings and Beliefs

L*et us be willing to release old hurts.*

—Martha Smock

As a psychic and a healer, I am often called upon to help clients release their negative or unresolved feelings or painful memories of the past (including memories of other lives). These are stored in our bodies until we resolve them. They are the roots of our physical problems, and their role should not be minimized. The unresolved emotional pain that we are storing inside affects our lives profoundly, threatening our health and our happiness.

Many of us are afraid or embarrassed to express our feelings, so instead, we stuff them deep down, where we hope they won't cause any trouble. We don't let our sadness or anger or fear or bitterness show. Doing so might make us feel vulnerable, out of control. We're afraid that someone is going to make fun of us.

Someone might call us a big baby or tell us that we are too sensitive, too emotional, or too dramatic.

What are your responses when someone starts talking to you about your feelings, your past, or your memories? Do you want to go smoke a pack of cigarettes or eat an entire chocolate cake? Maybe run off to the bingo parlor or the nearest casino? Park yourself on the couch with some junk food and turn on the tube? Maybe smoke a few joints or fix a few cocktails? Run out and do some shopping? I think I have had nearly every one of these responses when I have not wanted to feel my feelings.

What we may not realize is that stuffing our feelings, refusing to release them, just gives them more power.

Like many others, I have gone from one extreme to the other in dealing with my emotions. I used to believe my feelings would take control of my life if I allowed myself to experience them. I had so much anger that I was sure I would kill someone if I let it out. I had so much sadness, I thought I would cry a river if I ever shed a single tear. I also had a lot of guilt and shame. I didn't think that I could bear to look at all the reasons for these feelings. And so I tried my best to avoid them.

When we are in emotional pain, there are many ways to dull it. Most of us spend thousands of hours finding ways to hide from our pain. Distractions are everywhere. Even religion can be used as a distraction for avoiding our stored feelings and negative beliefs.

Internalizing Negative Feelings

Do I mean that every feeling you ever had, or that you never expressed, is sitting inside your body? No, not every feeling. I am talking about a particular category of feelings, mainly those

POSITIVE FEELINGS

bliss	happiness	passion
ecstasy	joy	satisfaction
excitement	love	sympathy
fulfillment	optimism	tenderness
gladness		

NEGATIVE FEELINGS

abandonment	failure	pride
aggression	fear	rage
agony	being forgotten	regret
anger	fright	rejection
anxiety	frustration	remorse
arrogance	greed	resentment
bashfulness	guilt	sadness
bewilderment	hate	shame
bitterness	helplessness	sheepishness
boredom	hopelessness	sorrow
being burdened	hostility	suspicion
confusion	inadequacy	terror
depression	isolation	being trapped
deprivation	jealousy	unimportance
desperation	limitedness	unwantedness
disappointment	loneliness	unworthiness
being discounted	misery	being used
doom	being withdrawn	panic
dread	paranoia	worry
envy	perplexity	

NEGATIVE BELIEFS ABOUT OURSELVES

I am:

unworthy	incompetent	incapable
unlovable	unwanted	unproductive
stupid	abandoned	undeserving
powerless	inadequate	trapped
guilty	inferior	burdensome
shameful	misunderstood	confused
bad	betrayed	weak
worthless	no good	unloved
alone	unattractive	
victimized	sinful	

Men/Women:

are inferior	have no power
create sorrow	abuse love
are undependable	abuse power
are hateful	abuse the opposite sex
like getting hurt	are victims
deserve pain	are weak

Family beliefs:

We will always be . . .

poor	misunderstood
stupid	disliked

associated with events in your life that have created or are reinforcing *negative* beliefs you have about yourself.

The words listed on the top of page 53 are often used to

describe *positive* situations or feelings. When these are felt and experienced in our lives they are a source of health. The words at the bottom of page 53 are often used to describe negative situations or feelings. These reinforce negative beliefs about yourself and keep you going in circles. As you go through this second list, you will probably find that you have a strong response to some of the words while you have little or no response to others. Make a note of which words elicit the strongest response.

These are the words that represent your negative belief system. As long as they are there, they can keep you stuck in a bad job or an abusive or unhappy relationship. They can be at the root of financial troubles or poor health. If you do nothing to change them, they will sit in your body and affect the rest of your life just as they affected your past.

The Hurt Inside

Now let's explore how all of this works. Let's say that I believe I am incapable of making a wise decision. Possibly one of my parents or a teacher said that to me once, or repeatedly, and I have held on to it, believing it to be true. Now, let's say a situation comes up in daily life when I need to make a decision. Panic or anger about making a wrong decision are two feelings that might come up immediately for me. I might also feel foolish, ashamed, guilty, depressed, or as if I were a failure. I may feel resentful toward the person or situation forcing me to make the decision.

The problem comes when I internalize all of these feelings and beliefs. I know this is happening because I get a tight stomach or maybe a sudden headache, a spastic colon, or a pain in the back of my neck. I go through this physical, mental, and emotional torture because I have this belief that I am incapable of making a wise decision. Furthermore, I don't feel comfortable expressing my negative feelings, such as anger, humiliation, shame, guilt, or sadness. So I just keep the whole mess inside. The belief is in there along with all the feelings I have surrounding that belief. Usually, it adds up to physical trouble somewhere in my body!

Here's another example: I have a belief that I am unlovable. No one would really love me for who I am. I do everything that I can to look lovable. I spend lots of money on my outside appearance. Every time I see someone I am interested in, I get anxious or even panicky. I pretend not be interested in him because I don't want him or anyone else to know how anxious I really am. He gets the message that I'm not interested in him, and so he leaves me alone. This reinforces my feelings of inadequacy, fear, and panic, as well as my belief that I am unlovable. I continue to feel alone, unloved, and misunderstood.

Feelings trigger the beliefs, and the beliefs trigger the negative feelings. Back and forth they go, like a Ping-Pong ball! Those beliefs sit inside, controlling our lives, affecting our worlds outside as well as within. As in the example above, they dictate our actions in the external world so that whatever occurs seem to validate our feelings.

If we are unable to express our feelings, they fester inside. As Woody Allen once said, "I don't get angry, I grow tumors instead."

Most people, I've found, intuitively understand this process. In an article published in the *Minneapolis Star Tribune,* a reporter interviewed grade-school children. He asked them how they handled stress. One eleven-year-old boy said, "I don't handle my worries. I just let them hurt me inside."

How insightful and how sad! The majority of us find it easier to store negative feelings than to go through the painful process of releasing them. Illness is a way to get to know ourselves.

It is a tool to change the course of our lives, a way to find freedom from the past. Pain, illness, and disease are our bodies' way of saying, "Help me to get unstuck. Help me to be free."

Releasing Negative Feelings

Sometimes, when we don't know what to do with our feelings, they can seem overwhelming. But how can you release your feelings in a way that makes you feel safe and that doesn't threaten those you are closest to? When feelings are buried deep, what is the best way to access them? Here are eight techniques I have used in my healing practice that you may find helpful:

1. **Write a letter.** If you find that you are really angry with another person or an institution, or you have certain feelings (hatred, resentment, sadness, etc.), write a letter. *You do not need to mail it!* The important thing is that you express exactly how you feel about that person or institution.

2. **Get support.** Share what you are feeling with a counselor or trusted friend. Sometimes we want someone to hear our feelings, though this is not always the person with whom we have a grievance.

3. **Role-play.** Place a chair in front of you, and pretend the person or institution is sitting in it. You might even tape his picture to the back of the chair. Say everything that you have ever wanted to say to this person about what he did to you. Don't worry about his feelings. Take care of your own! If this is someone who has abused you in some way, visualize giving back to the offender the shame, pain, and humiliation he gave to you. Don't worry about being impolite or behaving in an "inappropriate" way. Your first priority right now is you and your feelings.

4. **Let it out.** Sometimes, when I get really angry with someone

or something, I get into my car and drive to a place where I am alone. I yell and scream as loud as I need to. I say everything I need to, until I feel an inner release of the emotions. It really works!

Get a plastic bat (available at toy stores) and beat your bed, couch, or a strong pillow with it. Use something soft so you won't hurt your hands.

5. **Sing out loud.** Turn up the music and sing along with it, as loudly and as outrageously as you want! It's a great release! Play some of the oldies. Get those memories going. Sing!

6. **Shed some tears.** Put on sad music, go to a sentimental movie, wallow in old memories, whatever you need to do. Just let those tears out!

7. **Do something physical.** This could be dancing, jogging, running, swimming, walking fast, playing a sport, bicycling, or doing yard work. Running on the treadmill with classical music turned up really loud is what I love to do when I'm feeling stressed, overwhelmed, or angry. Anything physical really helps!

8. **Go outside.** Be out in nature. You will feel more grounded. You might work in a garden, mow the grass, rake the leaves, shovel snow, or go for a nature walk. If you can be outdoors and talk it out to the Universe—to the trees, birds, flowers, and rocks—it will really help to work that anxiety, fear, and anger out of your body.

Often, we hurt ourselves physically and emotionally because of unresolved feelings. This might include hitting, biting, cutting, or scratching yourself. It might include ramming your fist into the wall (hurting yourself more than the wall). It might include abusing yourself with your addictions—overeating, drinking, using drugs, overworking, spending too much money or money you don't have, or unnecessarily throwing yourself into situations that cause even more stress.

When it comes to self-punishment, most of us are very resourceful. Have you ever been exhausted but wouldn't accept it? You just kept on pushing and pushing and pushing. Or you may have sabotaged a job offer or a relationship that you really wanted but didn't feel you deserved. Again, you were punishing yourself because of unresolved feelings.

Time to Stop the Pain

One of the most important points in this book is that your stored inner pain, memories, and beliefs have hurt you enough. It is time to stop the pain! If you come up against feelings in the exercises in this chapter that you don't know what to do with, for goodness sake don't continue to punish yourself! There are ways to get those feelings out besides hitting, starving, or stuffing yourself; creating an illness; or acting them out in ways that will only cause more *dis-ease* in your life.

Start now to break those old, destructive, and hurtful patterns of taking unresolved pain out on yourself. After you've released some of your feelings, give yourself a break. Praise yourself for doing good work, for possibly closing a chapter in your life.

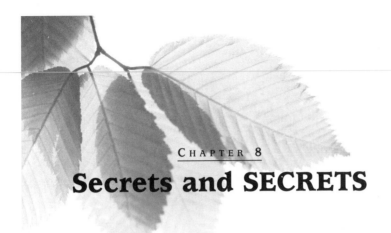

CHAPTER 8

Secrets and SECRETS

*W*hat happens to these secrets, these painful
memories that we continue to hold inside?
What happens to them?

—Echo Bodine

There are two kinds of secrets: those that are conscious and those that are unconscious. In this chapter we will examine both kinds and see how each affects our lives. First, let's take a look at how damaging consciously kept secrets can be.

A good friend of mine called recently. She was very upset because the youth pastor at her church had just committed suicide. She asked me if I would use my psychic abilities to see his soul clairvoyantly. She wanted some help in understanding why a popular, thirty-four-year-old pastor would lie beneath the exhaust pipes of his brand-new truck and take his own life. She said that this man had always been there for everyone. He seemed to love life and have everything going for him. These seem to be the standard remarks made about most people who commit suicide. While not everyone who has these traits commits suicide, it does seem to be the profile of people who never show they are in pain.

I was surprised that I was able to psychically tune in to this man so soon after his death. As soon as I closed my eyes, there he was in all of his pain. I saw, with the help of John, my spirit guide, that this man had been sexually abused as a young boy by two men close to him. One was his father; the other was his pastor. He grew up feeling very guilty and ashamed. He felt like a sinner, a very bad sinner. One of the major reasons he had gone into the clergy was to cleanse himself of his dirtiness. He never told anyone about being sexually abused; he was too ashamed. He felt that he was to blame for what had happened to him. Since becoming a pastor, he also had been entrusted with other people's secrets, and now he had more pain than he could bear. He wanted relief.

I asked John why the pastor had chosen suicide, instead of getting some professional help. John said that the man had been hopeful that getting out of his body and going to Heaven would rid him of his emotional pain. However, he found that once he got there, the pain was still with him. Also, he now felt guilty about the choice he had made to take his own life.

This young pastor had spent his entire life in the grips of a *consciously kept secret,* protecting two men he loved very much—men who had hurt him deeply.

As strange as it might seem, this man's choice was not unusual. Many clients I have seen over the years consciously choose to hang on to their pain. They remember the sexual, physical, or emotional abuse that has been done to them, and they know who the perpetrator was. But in no way are they ready to let their secret out. They tell me it was too embarrassing, too humiliating. They don't want to hurt the person who hurt them. They protect, and in some cases go so far as to defend, their victimizer rather than let the secret out.

What happens to these conscious secrets, these painful memories that we continue to hold inside? Do our memory banks store them safely and neatly for us, where they can do no harm to us or anyone else? Or is it possible that we store them somewhere in our bodies? And if so, could they possibly be the seeds of physical illness?

Do yourself a favor. Don't minimize the pain that was done to you. I believe that your secrets will chip away at the your physical body until you get some therapeutic help for the emotional pain and medical help for the physical pain. Release them and refuse to protect or defend those who may have caused you harm. Our secrets, particularly those secrets that are harboring pain, are all sitting inside our bodies.

What about those secrets in which you were the perpetrator, and someone else was the victim? Those also wreak havoc with your physical well-being. You may have stolen something from a friend or family member. You may have witnessed something hurtful done to you or someone else. You may have overheard someone telling a lie. You may have cheated someone. You may have abused a person or an animal, or had someone abuse you. You may think your secret has been cleverly tucked away, until it suddenly springs to mind the moment something triggers the memory. Until you release it—by talking about it openly to a confidant or in therapy—it will hide in your body, doing its physical damage.

Secrets We Keep from Ourselves

As I stated earlier, there are two kinds of secrets: those we keep from others (conscious) and those we keep from ourselves (unconscious). Secrets we keep from ourselves are difficult, but not impossible, to uncover. I believe that the body gives us many indications, often in the form of physical symptoms, which can help us get in touch with these secrets and let them out.

Your stored secrets are not necessarily the roots of all your physical problems, but they *are* going to cause some kind of physical or emotional problems. Your body does not need to be a dumping ground for other people's secrets or your own. It's vital to your health to summon all those secrets from their hiding places in your body.

To become aware of your unconscious secrets, begin by noting in your journal any recurring physical problems. Identifying the physical problems won't necessarily reveal your hidden secrets to you, so don't try to immediately figure them out. I was in denial for a long time before I admitted that there could be a connection between my physical problems and the secrets I was keeping.

To begin opening up to the secrets you are holding inside, just be still for a minute and focus on your body. What pains are you aware of right now? For what physical problems have you recently consulted a doctor? Think about the last five to ten years of your life. What were your recurring physical problems? If you were in an accident that resulted in long-term health issues, write these down as well.

When I thought about revealing secrets I was keeping inside, I feared getting into trouble or being called a "tattletale." Revealing secrets that you have held on to for years can be terrifying. You may find it easier to release your secrets in a safe setting, such as with a counselor or a trusted friend.

If you're still feeling stuck about disclosing your secrets, ask yourself why it's so scary. What do you think would happen if you did write down that secret? Would you be punished? Who would punish you? Why are you protecting yourself or the person whose secret you are holding? Don't get down on yourself if you're feeling afraid. Be gentle with yourself!

Sharing the secret means it is a secret no longer, and it is freed from your body forever. When the secret is no longer left inside, the burden of holding it in will be gone or greatly reduced, and along with it, the pain or illness it may have caused.

Journal Work

Exercise 1

Releasing Your Own Secrets

Begin this exercise by putting a line down the middle of a fresh page in your healing journal, making two columns. Label the first column "Conscious Secrets Stored Inside"; label the second column "Physical Aches/Pains."

Sitting in a comfortable position, take three or four deep breaths, breathing in clarity and blowing out tension and fear. Ask your body to bring to your conscious mind the secrets you are keeping inside. Write down in the first column of your journal, under "Conscious Secrets Stored Inside," whatever comes to mind. As the memories of these secrets surface, note how your body feels and record these in the column labeled "Physical Aches/Pains."

Exercise 2

Releasing Other People's Secrets

Divide a new page in your journal into two columns, this time labeling the first column "Other People's Secrets"; then label the second column, as before, "Physical Aches/Pains."

Record in the first column the secrets that other people have asked you to hold for them or which you feel you must keep for them. Notice how your body reacts as you bring each one to mind. Write these reactions down in the second column, "Physical Aches/Pains."

Take a break after completing this exercise. Go out and do something light and fun. Take a walk or a bike ride (see chapter 22 for more tips on how to have fun). This will help you to feel more grounded, better focused, centered, and unafraid.

Exercise 3

Getting Help from Your Inner Child

Put a pencil or crayon in your nondominant hand and ask your inner child what secrets it is holding inside. As the adult, comfort and reassure your inner child, as one would do with any child who is feeling afraid. Be loving and gentle. Be understanding and patient. Reassure your inner child that you will protect it so that no one will scold or punish it. Your inner child needs to know that it is safe. It may be necessary to repeat your reassurances several times before you begin to feel your body calming down.

Be sure to supply your inner child with plenty of paper for this exercise. When it finally begins letting the secrets out, they are likely to fill up many pages.

Remember that when your inner child begins to express itself, the critical parent is likely to jump in and be critical or simply deny that any of it is true. You may wish to record these critical parent comments as you go along.

Exercise 4

Creating a Safe Place

When you have completed the above exercises, dialogue with your inner child and ask what it now needs to feel safe. Do what you can to create an emotional atmosphere of safety and love in your mind.

After completing this work, sit back, take a few deep breaths, and relax. Read these words to yourself:

I am an adult now.

I can protect myself.

I will not let any more pain happen to me or my inner child.

Just sit and feel the safety of these words and their promise. Know that what you have said is true.

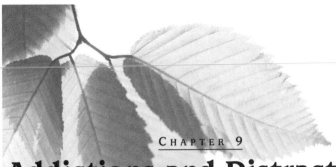

CHAPTER 9

Addictions and Distractions

*W*e cannot heal our addictive mind while it is entrenched in fear and conflict. It would be like trying to get out of a Chinese finger puzzle: the harder you pull, the tighter it becomes.

—Lee Jampolsky

One of the ways we deal with our unresolved pain, secrets, feelings, and negative beliefs is through addictions and distractions. My own experience of growing up in an addicted family can perhaps provide some insights into how this works. On the outside, I appeared to be super-responsible—a peacemaker, a perfectionist, a caretaker, a leader, serious-minded, confident, rigid, and in control. On the inside, I felt lonely, inadequate, afraid, confused, angry, hurt, guilty, ashamed, forever unsatisfied, afraid of making mistakes, and out of control. I acted the opposite of what I felt on the inside, not wanting people to know how inadequate I believed I was. I wanted to appear confident and strong!

By the time I was nineteen, alcohol seemed to have become the perfect solution to all my inner pain and the contradictions that I was living. This occurred despite my childhood oath that I would never drink. At age eighteen, I didn't think that "just one drink" could hurt. I was on a date and didn't want to appear anything less than "cool." When my date asked me what I wanted to drink, I said, "Whatever you are having." I became very drunk and blacked out. The next day I couldn't remember a thing.

From that day on, I never drank in moderation. I drank straight alcohol so that I could become numb and not feel all of my internal pain and conflicts. Alcohol gave me the confidence I had never known. Also, it was a great excuse for being obnoxious; it allowed me to release all of my anger and rage. I couldn't drink every day, since my body would get too sick. But I would get drunk at least twice a week. When I wasn't drinking, I was thinking about it—always preoccupied with escaping from reality and my feelings.

At the age of twenty-three, I was rear-ended in a car accident. This turned out to be the beginning of the end of my drinking career and the beginning of my addiction to prescription drugs. My neck, back, and upper arms had been injured in the accident. An orthopedic surgeon prescribed Valium to relax my muscles. He also prescribed Percodan, a powerful narcotic, and a painkiller, Talwin. A neurologist put me on Fiorinal, also a painkiller, for all of the headaches that I was experiencing. Despite all the physical pain I was in, this was an addict's heaven! On days when I had a hangover, I could take a bunch of pills and they would make my emotional pain so much easier to bear. On days when I mixed alcohol and pills, I felt even better! Throughout my alcoholism and pill addiction, I also acted out with other addictions. I used food to ease my pain (more on that later). Men and relationships were also an addiction. I was forever looking outside myself for a way to feel better.

It was a frightening, frantic lifestyle. All of that unresolved pain was constantly trying to surface. Instead of looking at the issues, I just stayed high. I was terrified of my emotions. I frequently thought about suicide.

Then, at the age of twenty-four, two weeks after the death of a very close friend, I hit bottom physically, mentally, emotionally, and spiritually. I could not go on living in the pain anymore. I joined Alcoholics Anonymous (AA). This was the beginning of my healing journey.

At AA, and in Al-Anon five years later, I worked the twelve steps to recovery.

The Effects of Addiction

Addicts minimize ("I only had one drink"), rationalize ("If you had my job, you'd drink, too!"), and deny that there is any problem. This is true for all addictions, not just addiction to alcohol. At the end of this chapter is a list of the questions used by Alcoholics Anonymous, Overeaters Anonymous, and Sex Addicts Anonymous. These will help you determine if you are covering up your internal pain through addiction(s). For those of you who may wonder if you have a gambling problem, substitute the word "gambling" for alcohol. If you are concerned that you have a drug problem, substitute the word "drugs" for alcohol, and so on.

I know the devastating effect of chemicals. I was always sick from taking them—regardless of whether or not I was hung-over. I had headaches and digestive and colon problems. If you are a practicing addict, your body is suffering from abuse. The toxins from your pill of choice can bring disastrous results: high blood pressure, gall bladder disease, strokes, diabetes, uterine cancer, or infant mortality. (This list comes from *Overeaters Anonymous, A Disease of the Body,* p. 90.)

Alcoholics and drug addicts can add to that list: liver disease; pancreatic problems; blood, stomach, colon, and kidney malfunctioning; brain dysfunctions; sleep and sexual disorders; paralysis; malnutrition; night blindness; infectious diseases; skin diseases; anemia; reproductive disorders; menstrual problems; infertility; repeated miscarriages; fetal alcohol syndrome; respiratory disorders; heart problems; and psychiatric disorders. This list goes on and on.

Once you have joined a recovery program, don't think for a second that you're "home free." The real work is only beginning. But the reward, you'll later realize, will be worth it, including freedom from the physical, emotional, and internalized pain that began your addictions. If you choose the other path—if you try to rationalize or deny your addiction—the consequences may be dire.

Connor, a man in his early forties with a four-pack-a-day smoking habit, came to me for a series of healings for his chronic cough. He hadn't been to a doctor because he assumed he would just be given a prescription, and the problem would not really be addressed. Furthermore, he was a recovering alcoholic and didn't want to risk becoming addicted to a prescription drug.

Connor also told me that he was a heavy gambler. When I looked inside him psychically, his lungs were as black as night. I saw two smokestacks filled to the brim with smoke and toxins. His heart looked very stressed and broken. I saw an image of a woman who had broken his heart, and he was still hanging on to her and the relationship, too, even though it looked as if it had been a long time since they had been together.

Next, I saw the physical result of his addiction: his body, riddled with a lifetime of pain and resentment. The spirits told me that the man's smoking and gambling were his way of distracting himself from the pain. But it had clearly taken its toll.

After three healing sessions, Connor's cough appeared to be getting worse. I believed that this was a result of the healing energy releasing the smoke and toxins from his lungs. The healings felt like a losing battle and he needed to go see a doctor in spite of his fears.

Medical tests revealed that he had cancer throughout his body. He died within a year of his first visit to me. Connor's case is a grim reminder of how important it is to clear out all those unresolved feelings and negative beliefs we have about ourselves.

The Addictive Cycle

Addiction isn't a one-trick pony. In many of the different twelve-step groups that I have attended, members are frequently recovering from multiple addictions. If you're an addict, your addiction may surface in multiple forms and with multiple substances. It's also a very common occurrence for an addict to go from one addiction to another—for example, to stop using alcohol and become an overeater, or to stop overeating and become a compulsive shopper.

Addicts are also frequently plagued by unresolved emotional pain, negative personal beliefs, and low self-esteem. These are the things that keep the addictive cycle going. Until we completely surrender the pain and begin a new way of living, we are fighting a losing battle. Addictions work in a very cunning manner. If you are in therapy, thinking that you are working on your issues, and then getting high after your sessions, you are really just going in circles!

Defeating your addictive behaviors begins by admitting you need help. Examine the questionnaires on these pages. If you find yourself described in any of them, ask the Universe to give you the strength and courage that you need to make the necessary changes. You can break this cycle of insanity and start feeling good *now!*

DISTRACTIONS

Distractions are another form of addiction, and just as dangerous. Distractions are anything we do to distract ourselves from our feelings. We might not think of these activities as addictive; after all, how bad can it be to turn on the TV, sit in front of the computer, work nonstop, travel, join a committee, adopt a pet, or play bingo? But if we do these things to excess—if we are *compelled* to do them because we are using them as a means of escaping ourselves, then yes, they are addictive behaviors.

In the age of the Internet, there are many seductive means of escape—into chat rooms or on X-rated web sites, selling or buying on eBay, or watching videos or movies. Countless hours spent in front of the computer screen may be a sign that you are trying to escape something. If you recognize these patterns in your life, make sure they are not a cover-up for addressing lingering issues. The main thing to remember is that from every form of addiction, recovery is possible.

ARE YOU AN ALCOHOLIC?

To answer this question, ask yourself the following questions and answer them as honestly as you can:

1. Do you lose time from work due to drinking?
2. Is drinking making your home life unhappy?
3. Do you drink because you are shy with other people?
4. Is drinking affecting your reputation?
5. Have you ever felt remorse after drinking?
6. Have you gotten into financial difficulties as a result of your drinking?
7. Do you turn to lower companions and an inferior environment when drinking?
8. Does your drinking make you careless about your family's welfare?
9. Has your ambition decreased since drinking?
10. Do you crave a drink at a definite time of day?
11. Do you want to drink the next morning?
12. Does drinking cause you to have difficulty in sleeping?
13. Has your efficiency decreased since you started drinking?
14. Is drinking jeopardizing your job or business?
15. Do you drink to escape from worries or trouble?
16. Do you drink alone?
17. Have you ever had a complete loss of memory as a result of drinking?
18. Has your physician ever treated you for drinking?
19. Do you drink to build up your self-confidence?

20. Have you ever been to a hospital or institution on account of drinking?

If you answered yes to any one of the questions, there is a chance that you may be an alcoholic.

If you answered yes to any two, the chances are that you are an alcoholic.

If you answered yes to three or more, you are definitely an alcoholic.

An alcoholic is anyone whose drinking disrupts business or interferes with family or social life. An alcoholic cannot stop drinking, even though she may want to do so.

THE "20 QUESTIONS" OF
SEXUAL ADDICTS ANONYMOUS (SAA)

The following are some questions to ask yourself to determine if you may be sexually addicted and to evaluate your need for the SAA program:

1. Do you use sex to escape from worries or troubles or to "relax"? Do you use sex to hide from other issues in your life?

2. Are you preoccupied with your sexual fantasies?

3. Do you usually feel compelled to have sex again and again within a short period of time?

4. Do you find it difficult to be friends with other men or women because of thoughts or fantasies about being sexual with them?

5. Has your sexual behavior made you feel scared or "different"—somehow alienating you from other people?

6. Have you repeatedly tried to stop what you believed was wrong in your sexual behavior? Is your sexual behavior often inconsistent with your values?

7. Are you concerned about how much time you spend in sexual fantasies?

8. Does your pursuit of sex interfere with your normal sexual relationship with your spouse or lover?

9. Have you ever made promises to yourself or to your regular sexual partner to change, limit, or control your sexual behavior, attitudes, or fantasies, and then broken these promises over and over again?

10. Do you find it almost impossible to have sex without resorting to certain kinds of fantasies or memories of "unique" scenarios?

11. Have you found yourself compelled by your desires to the point where your regular sexual partner has resisted?

12. Has your desire for sex driven you to associate with persons or to spend time in places you would not normally choose?

13. Have you ever felt you'd be better off if you didn't need to give in to your sexual obsessions or compulsions?

14. Do you frequently feel remorse, guilt, or shame after a sexual encounter? Do you frequently want to get away from this sex partner after having sex?

15. Have your family, friendships, job, or school work suffered because of your sexual obsessions or activities? Do you take time from them to engage in sex or look for sexual adventures?

16. Have you been arrested or nearly arrested because of your sexual behavior? Have your sexual activities jeopardized your life goals?

17. Do your sexual activities include the risk of contracting disease or being maimed or killed by a violent sexual partner?

18. Has compulsive masturbation become a substitute for the kind of sexual relationship you want with your spouse or lover?

19. Does a periodic inability to have sex abate or disappear only when you engage in what you would judge to be illicit sexual activity?

20. Do your sexual behavior or fantasies ever make you feel hopeless, anxious, depressed, or suicidal?

Many people have answered yes to some of these questions, and as a result sought help through the SAA program.

ARE YOU A COMPULSIVE OVEREATER?

1. Do you eat when you're not hungry?

2. Do you go on eating binges for no apparent reason?

3. Do you have feelings of guilt and remorse after overeating?

4. Do you give too much time and thought to food?

5. Do you look forward with pleasure and anticipation to the moments when you can eat alone?

6. Do you plan these secret binges ahead of time?

7. Do you eat sensibly in front of others and make up for it when you are alone?

8. Is your weight affecting the way you live your life?

9. Have you tried to diet for a week (or longer), only to fall short of your goal?

10. Do you resent the advice of others who tell you to "use a little will power" to stop overeating?

11. Despite evidence to the contrary, have you continued to assert that you can diet "on your own" whenever you wish?

12. Do you crave eating at a definite time, day or night, other than mealtimes?

13. Do you eat to escape from worries or trouble?

14. Has your physician ever treated you for being overweight?

15. Does your food obsession make you or others unhappy?

How did you score? If you answered yes to three or more of these questions, it is probable that you have a compulsive eating problem or are well on the way to having one.

The Courage to Heal

If you are a practicing addict of anything, my heart goes out to you. My prayer for you is that this miserable nightmare in which you are living goes away soon and that you can set off on the road to recovery. You deserve the best in life, but you will never experience it until you learn to heal the inner wounds that are causing your pain.

The fact that there are so many support groups in communities throughout the United States indicates not only that help is available to you whenever you choose to reach out but also that you are not alone. Thousands of people every year enter twelve-step programs in order to seek freedom from one addiction or another, whether it's alcohol, food, sex, or any of a wide range of prescription or street drugs.

Perhaps one of the most important things we have to learn on any healing journey is that we are responsible for taking the first step. The healing begins when we finally decide it is time to look inside ourselves and confront the pain we are hiding inside. As challenging as that task may seem, I would like to assure you that it is far easier, and less painful, than continuing to live a life of addiction.

Inner Work

Take the time to make notes in your healing journal about any of your findings in this chapter. If the subject of addiction did not seem to apply to you, you might want to note how it perhaps did apply to someone in your life, from either the past or the present. Note any thoughts you have about this person.

While not everyone has an obvious addiction, or even a habit that causes harm or limits their lives, we all have ways of distracting ourselves from the things that are bothering us. Note any techniques you have for distracting yourself or for getting away from uncomfortable feelings. Simply take note of these without judging them.

If you feel that you are caught up in addictive behavior of any kind, or are involved with a person who is, realize that this issue is part of your healing. Start this healing by entering a support group or twelve-step program (more on this in chapter 19). Al-Anon and Codependents Anonymous are great places to begin. Contact the local chapter of the program that applies to you or call the Alcoholics Anonymous Intergroup Office nearest you for information. Use a page in your journal to record names of organizations, their meeting times, where they meet, and the names and phone numbers of resource people whom you may discover along the way.

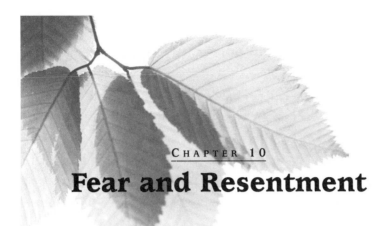

CHAPTER 10

Fear and Resentment

Our society has tremendous prohibitions against feeling too much. We are afraid to feel too much fear, hurt, sadness, or anger; and oftentimes we are also afraid to feel too much love, passion, or joy! And we're definitely afraid of our natural sensuality and sexuality.

—Shakti Gawain

Fear is like an evil ghost. We know that it's there; we pretend it isn't, and we're afraid to do anything about it. So it just takes up residence wherever it feels like and goes on haunting us. But there is good fear and bad fear and it can be helpful to be able to tell one from the other.

Healthy fear gives us a sense of when something really isn't safe. It warns us of danger. Otherwise, we might all be jumping off cliffs or walking through Central Park alone at night. The good news is that healthy fear isn't going to hurt us. It protects us from getting hurt.

Negative fear, however, can cripple us. It shows up in the body as a very icy-cold energy. Oftentimes, if a person is carrying a great deal of fear, I can feel about five inches of a thick coldness that either sits in certain areas of the body or completely envelops it.

Suzanne, a young woman in her early thirties, came to me for a healing that had to do with her fear around love. There were cold spots throughout her body. She had just fallen in love but had many negative messages inside: her parents' bitter divorce; disappointing past relationships; painful, past-life memories concerning love, of which she wasn't conscious but were there nonetheless. She felt that her new love was right for her in many ways, and she did not want anything to interfere with this relationship's potential. Yet, fear was holding her back. She discovered that she would only be able to go forward and let the relationship unfold if she learned to release herself from the negative images of the past that were stored in her body.

Fear and Physical Pain

Many years ago, I sat in a hospital, waiting to undergo my fourth surgery in two years. It was to be the second surgery on my colon. I was very upset that I was back in the hospital and that I was still in pain after three other attempts to correct the problem. Why was I going through all of this? Was it some karmic debt from another lifetime? I felt very frustrated that I couldn't see for myself what was going on. Here I was, a psychic who had helped many other people understand why they went through similar situations, yet I couldn't see what was going on with me!

My mom called a medicine man she knew in South Dakota and asked him if he could see why I was back in this same predicament. He called me at the hospital the day before the surgery to tell me he'd had a vision of my colon being full of fear. He said that I had been storing in my body all of my fearful memories since childhood. I had to work on releasing all the fears stored in my colon if I ever wanted it to work properly.

When I hung up the phone, I felt overwhelmed. Where in the world to begin? I had hoped that he would give me some magical words; then I could pack my bags and go home. I felt so alone and so afraid. There was a part of me that knew he was right, even though intellectually I wasn't yet convinced that stored emotions could have such a devastating effect on my body.

I had the surgery. The doctor corrected the physical problem by removing thirteen inches of twisted intestines. I knew intuitively that I needed to work on surrendering my fears rather than holding on to them. I did not want to have any more surgery or any more pain. I wanted to heal.

Facing the Fear

It took some time for me to be honest with myself. My first reaction when the medicine man had told me the problem was fear was to try my best to dispute the facts: "No way do I have any fear. I am tough. I can handle anything." The truth was that I was very fearful despite the fact that I was handling things. It took me a long time to be willing to see this.

I believe that all of us, especially those of us who are traveling a spiritual path, eventually need to face our fears. We can't in all honesty say that we're faith-filled, if in fact we are fear-filled. If there is an inner conflict between faith and fear, we must work on resolving it. Emmanuel says, "People have to deal with fear because it is one of the greatest denials of the reality of God" (*Emmanuel's Book*, p. 164).

It has taken me a while, but I think that I have identified most of my fears. I find now that when I get a pain I am usually able to identify the cause as something in my life that's making me feel afraid. I know it's time for me to surrender those fears once again. I would like you to start becoming aware of what your own fears may be, so you can write them down in your journal.

Resentment

Resentment, like fear, has the ability to make our lives miserable. Fortunately, both are totally under our control. *Webster's* defines resentment as taking "strong exception to what is thought to be unjust, interfering, insulting, critical." To me, it's remembering a hurt that has been done to me and not wanting to let it go—harboring angry or hateful feelings. Sometimes resentment means scheming and plotting ways to get back at the person who hurt us.

As a healer, I have seen that resentment can be the root cause of many physical problems. When we continue to hold on to the injustices other people have inflicted upon us, resentment builds inside us, causing serious damage to our bodies. If you make a statement to yourself, such as "I will never forget what so-and-so did to me," you are consciously storing that memory in your body, along with the bitterness and hatred. Our resentments become bitter stories that grow with the passing of time.

A client named Eric came to see me because of his hearing difficulties. He told me that one day he had been hunting with his best friend when the gun went off in close proximity to his ear. He had been having trouble with his hearing ever since.

The first time that Eric told me this story, the mishap seemed quite unintentional. But I found that each time he repeated it, the details of the story changed. Once, when he came for his appointment, he was in a particularly bad mood; nothing had gone right for him at work that day, and he'd come home to house full of angry, unruly kids. This time, when he told me the story, he revealed that his friend had been trying to kill him!

Was this true? Or was Eric embellishing the facts? In terms of his healing, the only thing that really mattered was that he forgive his friend and let the story go. Once he released his resentment, I told him his ear would begin to heal.

Many people don't know any other way to get attention or sympathy or love than to share their stories about how they've been hurt. They repeat their stories over and over again, telling anyone and everyone who'll listen all the details about "who done them wrong."

This is a tough way to live. Every day, people intentionally or unintentionally hurt us. Most often it's unintentional. Each time a hurt comes our way, we have the choice to either let it go or hang on to it and store it away until we can get back at them. We believe we will be able to rest only when we feel that justice has been served. But as quickly as justice is served in one case, another injustice is there to take its place, because resentment has become a habit.

Letting Go

If you've been slighted, hurt, or injured, your body will store your own story of injustice so you can tell it over and over again. Somehow, we think that if we never forgive and forget the people who hurt us, that *they* will suffer the punishment. The simple truth is that we're the ones who end up crippled with arthritis, back pain, headaches, cancer, or whatever. The resentment is killing us, not the people we find so hard to forgive.

One characteristic of resentment is that it is often not as obvious to us as it is to others. Instead of waiting for an apology, all we have to do is express our feelings to whomever has hurt us, and healing can be instantaneous.

Rosalie came to me in search of healing for her sprained ankle, which was the result of a freak accident. A male friend who had been staying with her was late for a job interview and found that his car was out of gas. He asked Rosalie if she could drive him there. In her rush to get ready, she tripped and fell, spraining her ankle. Not only did her friend not offer to help her, he left her in pain and rushed off to hail a taxi.

It was now several months later, and still Rosalie's ankle would not heal. It was only through a psychic reading that I learned that she was subconsciously holding on to her resentment. I told her that what she was really hanging on to was the hope that her friend would one day acknowledge the role he had played in what had happened and apologize for leaving her in pain. As soon as she was able to release her resentment by offering her friend forgiveness, Rosalie's ankle started to heal.

If you are still hanging on to negative feelings about something that happened to you a long time ago, these feelings are being held inside of you where they can do damage to your health! Don't minimize these feelings. Let go of the resentment you may be holding inside.

When We Have Hurt Others

Another side of the resentment issue that is not so pleasant to look at has to do with the pain we have caused others. The eighth step of AA's twelve-step program is making a list of all persons we have harmed and becoming willing to make amends to them all. Step 9 is making direct amends to such people wherever possible, except when doing so would injure them or others.

What does it mean to make amends? *Webster's* says: "To correct, to improve; to change or revise." It's not only apologizing for the hurt that we have caused others, but it's changing our future behavior toward that person. The apology isn't much good if we apologize for something and then turn right around and do it again! What is most important of all is changing our own behavior.

It can be helpful to ask God, the Universe, or whatever is your concept of a Higher Power to help you be willing to acknowledge those hurts that you have caused others. I know that acknowledging that there are people you have harmed is not pleasant, but it's a vital part of the healing journey. Remember, this has nothing to do with who's right and who's wrong. Don't get caught in the trap of who hurt whom more. Taking care of your unfinished business is *for your sake, your healing*. It has nothing to do with your concept of justice.

One final thought: in making amends to the people you have harmed, be very careful not to injure anybody in the process. When considering making amends, ask yourself if the amendment you are thinking about is going to make the other person feel better. If it may cause the other more harm, don't do it. While the purpose of making amends is to clean out all the old guilt and shame, as well as to wipe the slate clean, it is not to be done at another's expense! In many cases, *the very best way we can make amends is to forgive ourselves for the harm we caused.*

Journal Work

Exercise 1

List Your Fears

In your journal, make a list of the things, people, or situations you fear. List every fear that comes into your mind, no matter how small it may seem. List it even though you may think it is silly or unjustified. Remember, you don't have to share this list with anyone. When you've finished making your list, read it over. As you read, are you aware of pain anywhere in your body? If so, jot it down next to the fear.

The purpose here is to start getting these fears out of your body and down on paper where they can do you no harm.

Exercise 2

List Your Resentments

Divide one or more pages in your journal into three columns. Label the first one "Name of Person/Organization"; label the middle one "What They Did to Me"; label the third one "My Feelings Then and Now."

When you have finished with your own list, ask a close friend or relative whether she knows of any other resentments you might be carrying around. Often, we forget details from our own stories. We may have shared our "war stories" with friends who will remind us how angry or resentful we were at the time. Our parents can remind us of resentments we may have been carrying around since childhood. If you discover more resentments, add them to your list.

Exercise 3

Make Amends

Divide one or more journal pages into three columns again, this time labeling them, respectively: "People I Have Harmed," "What I Did to Them," and "How I Will Make Amends."

Now fill in the blank spaces. Remember my earlier caution about making amends only if they will do no harm. And remember, too, that sometimes healing begins by finding it in your heart to forgive yourself.

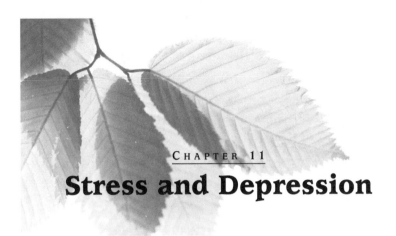

Stress and Depression

Your symptoms may not be in your head, but the power to get rid of them may well be.

—Stuart Berger, MD

Sometimes stress and depression go together like a hand in a glove. But not always. So we'll address them separately in this chapter.

What is stress? Stress is your body's reaction to any conflicting or excessive demands placed upon it. Have you ever gone to your doctor with some physical problem, only to have him say: "I can't find anything wrong. It must be stress"? The statement, "it must be stress," somehow minimizes any physical or emotional problem you may be having. There's also an unspoken message that implies that you should just "cope better" with your life.

Do you ever stop and think how much you go through each day? Each day as you perform your routines, interact with other people, and make decisions for your life and that of others, challenges face you at every turn. Your mind is constantly engaged in thinking through the moment or racing ahead to plan for what must be done next. Your feelings are always operating at some level, too, whether or not you are aware of them.

In the course of a day, there are bill collectors, health emergencies, deaths, accidents, holidays, unexpected work or school assignments, traffic delays, schedules running behind due to circumstances beyond our control, phone lines busy, computers shutting down, threatening mail, the school nurse calling to say that your child needs to come home, long lines at the checkout counter, a flat tire or other car trouble, the bus breaking down, changes in the company management, appointments getting canceled or changed.

Most of us do not realize how much stress we place on our bodies and minds each day. We take life's demands with a grain of salt and scarcely even notice our daily challenges until we become completely exhausted or ill.

The only way for our body to get our attention when it is feeling burned out or stressed to the limit is to send some kind of signal that something is wrong.

I took a stress management class to learn how to cope with stress. In the class, we listed the physical symptoms people experience as a result of stress. Here is a list of the health problems we came up with:

aches	diarrhea	hyperventilation
alcohol abuse	disassociation	impotence
anxiety attacks	drug abuse	insomnia
back pains	eating disorders	jaw tightness
bladder problems	eye strain	cancer
manic-depressive	over-stimulation	canker sores
syndrome	headaches	paranoia
fatigue	colitis	heart attacks

prostate problems   constipation   hemorrhoids

smoking   death   herpes

stroke   diabetes   hypertension

sexual dysfunction   vaginal infection

RATING YOUR BURNOUT LEVEL

Often, we don't even recognize the early signs of burnout when they occur. When we're in the middle of it, we're too depleted to see what's happening to us. The following test was derived from the work of Dr. Herbert J. Freudenberger, author of a book entitled *Burn Out: The High Cost of High Achievement.* Freudenberger coined the term "burnout."

The Test

Start by looking back over the past six months. Mentally note if there have been any changes at the office, in the family, in your social situations. Have you noticed any changes in yourself or in the way you have been relating to the world around you? Give yourself about thirty seconds to think about each of the following fifteen questions. Then rate yourself on each point according to a scale of 1 to 5, with 5 meaning that you've experienced the most change, 1 meaning the least.

1. Have you noticed that you tire more easily lately? Do you generally feel fatigued rather than energetic?

2. Have people begun telling you that you don't look so good lately?

3. Does it seem that you are working harder and accomplishing less and less?

4. Are you increasingly cynical or disenchanted?

5. Do you experience sudden spells of sadness you can't explain?

6. Are you becoming forgetful about appointments and deadlines, or are you losing the car keys or misplacing personal objects?

7. Are you becoming increasingly irritable or short-tempered? Or are you feeling more disappointed than usual in the people around you?

8. Are you visiting with close friends and family members less often?

9. Are you so busy that you can't find the time to do routine things such as making phone calls, reading reports, or sending out your Christmas cards?

10. Do you have nagging physical complaints such as aches and pains, headaches, or a lingering cold or sinus infection?

11. Do you feel disoriented at the end of the day when you have completed your usual activities?

12. Are you missing a sense of joy in your life?

13. Have you lost your sense of humor about yourself?

14. Has sexual activity become more trouble than it's worth?

15. Do you feel you have very little to say to people?

Tally up your total points and roughly rate yourself on the burnout scale below. Keep in mind that this is only a rough approximation, useful as a guide for reducing stress in your life. Don't be alarmed if you get a high stress rating. But don't ignore it, either. Burnout is reversible, no matter how far along it is. But higher ratings suggest that the sooner you start being kinder to yourself, the better.

The Burnout Scale

0–25   Okay. You are handling stress well.

26–35   Pay attention. There are areas of stress you should be reducing or eliminating.

36–50   Caution. You could be a candidate for burnout.

51–65   Trouble. You are burning out.

Over 65 Danger! You are definitely in a dangerous place, one that could threaten your physical and mental well-being.

It is important to find a way to express the pressures and stresses we feel in our lives. Talk about them, whatever they may be. Do you have someone in your family or a close friend who is seriously ill or perhaps even dying? That is a major stress for everyone concerned. Have you got troubles on the job? Problems in a relationship? With your children? Health issues yourself? Roommate problems? How about your finances? Maybe you've got a new baby in the house, or a new pet? Even situations that bring joy can cause extra stress.

We all tend to minimize stress, and it's time to stop doing that! We need to acknowledge its impact on us, mentally and physically. Don't just tell yourself you've got to learn how to cope better.

Stress Relief

Healing begins by taking note of the impact stress may be having on our lives. This means not just noticing the stressors themselves, but also our reaction to them. A customer may scream and yell at you because you messed up the order, but how you react to his anger is up to you. If you acknowledge your mistake or defend it without getting uptight, you are far less likely to hold negative feelings in your body. Finishing up business is a wonderful way to minimize the day's stress and prevent it from spilling over from one day into the next.

I would like to suggest that from now on, at the end of each day, you take five minutes and review what has occurred. Are you still holding stress from the day's events in your body? Exactly what happened to cause you to feel stressful? Write it down in your journal. If you don't take stress to bed with you, you will be able to make a fresh start each day.

The concept of living your life one day at a time is a good one. In our Western culture, we are used to jumping ahead; we want to anticipate, to know what's coming around each bend. We want to plan. We want to be ready. We hate not being in control.

Giving up control is one of the strongest ways to promote healing. Try it. Life will become much easier, I promise you!

Depression

In my younger years, I suffered from a manic-depressive disorder. That's what the psychological tests have always called it. I had extreme mood swings. When I was manic, I would feel on top of the world. I would talk a lot. I'd feel like shouting or screaming in delight, but there wasn't anything to shout or scream about. You know that feeling when you're small and waiting for Santa Claus or your birthday party or a trip to your favorite amusement park? You feel like you're going to jump out of your skin, you're so excited.

That's what the manic side of my cycle felt like, only more intense. You literally feel like the top of your head is going to fly off with excitement. The good news is that it doesn't last long. The bad news is that you come down. Way down. You crash into the depression part of manic depression. There is nothing in my life that I ever dreaded more than the onset of depression.

For all of you who suffer from depression, who have possibly even considered suicide, I hope you will hear these words. Depression is treatable! You don't have to be a victim of this disease for the rest of your life!

Today as I was trying to prepare myself mentally to write about my old nemesis, I was reading through *Depression and Its Treatment* by John H. Griest, MD, and James W. Jefferson, MD. I wanted to refresh my memory of the pain that I once thought I would never be able to forget. In the chapter on "What Is Depression," the authors include a patient's description of her depression. As I was reading her story, flashes of old memories came to me. Old pain, frustration, loneliness. That incredible despair that no one seems to understand unless they have been there. The helplessness. The hopelessness and emptiness. The aloneness of not being able to describe that inner desperation. A past, present, and future that all feel heavy, bleak, and useless.

Reading the story made me feel very afraid. I didn't want to write about depression. I wanted to forget about it and go on to something else. I felt really anxious inside. I was afraid that if I thought about it too much, it would find me again after these many years of being free of it.

I got out my vacuum cleaner and began furiously vacuuming my house. I didn't feel much relief. I decided to mow my grass. I was observing myself go through all of this. One part of me was saying, "Are you crazy? It's ninety degrees outside and you have to get this chapter written!" But there was another part of me that had to get away from my desk and do something physical.

I mowed my lawn as if someone were chasing me. I had headphones on with the music blasting. Memories flooded my mind of past depressions. I felt anger about having gone through all of them. I felt sorry for myself. I remembered all the times I had tried to explain to people how I felt and realized how futile it was to even try. This always made me feel crazier and more alone than ever.

Each time a bout would come, I weighed the pros and cons of suicide.

At the same time, I always wondered why this was happening to me. Nothing specific seemed to trigger the onset of a depression. Yet slowly it would creep in, and then after a time, sometimes after days, weeks, or months, it would just stop. Today, I believe that all the pain and memories, unresolved issues, feelings, and beliefs sitting inside would just overwhelm my body. Then, in a sense, I would break down and get depressed.

Different therapists suggested various medications over the years, but because of my former addiction to pills I was very leery of taking anything. My AA sponsor worked with me on the depression. He, too, had suffered from manic-depressive disorder. When I would begin going into the manic high, he would tell me over and over, "Bring those highs down and those lows up. Don't let yourself go so high or get so low." It did help, even though it was difficult to do because when someone is depressed, she doesn't care. It was tough to fight that apathy.

If you suspect that you suffer from depression, whether it's every day or only periodically, I suggest that you take the inventory on page 97. If you find you do suffer from depression, seek professional help. Don't try to fix it on your own. If you could, you would have done so by now! You're not an expert. Even if you are an expert and are suffering from it, get some help! *You do not have to live with depression.*

Treatment for Depression

If you are diagnosed with depression, you won't necessarily be put on drugs, but if so, there are many new drugs that don't have all of the side effects old medications had. In fact, most people who have serious chronic depression are able to work with a psychiatrist to get exactly the right medication, one that will have few or no side effects whatsoever.

If you are not getting what you need to change your depressed state (and I'm not talking about getting stoned on tranquilizers to

BECK DEPRESSION INVENTORY (BDI)

This questionnaire contains groups of statements. Please read each group of statements carefully. Then pick out the one statement in each group which best describes the way you have been feeling the *past week, including today.* Circle the number beside the statement you picked. If several statements in the group seem to apply equally, circle the highest number. Be sure to read all the statements in each group before making your choice.

1.0 I do not feel sad.

   1 I feel sad.

   2 I am sad all the time and I can't snap out of it.

   3 I am so sad or unhappy that I can't stand it.

2.0 I am not particularly discouraged about the future.

   1 I feel discouraged about the future.

   2 I feel I have nothing to look forward to.

   3 I feel that the future is hopeless and that things cannot improve.

3.0 I do not feel like a failure.

   1 I feel I have failed more than the average person.

   2 As I look back on my life, all I can see is a lot of failures.

   3 I feel I am a complete failure as a person.

4.0 I get as much satisfaction out of things as I used to.

   1 I don't enjoy things the way I used to.

   2 I don't get real satisfaction out of anything anymore.

   3 I am dissatisfied or bored with everything.

5.0 I don't feel particularly guilty.

  1 I feel guilty a good part of the time.

  2 I feel quite guilty most of the time.

  3 I feel guilty all the time.

6.0 I don't feel I am being punished.

  1 I feel I may be punished.

  2 I expect to be punished.

  3 I feel I am being punished.

7.0 I don't feel disappointed in myself.

  1 I am disappointed in myself.

  2 I am disgusted with myself.

  3 I hate myself.

8.0 I don't feel I am any worse than anybody else.

  1 I am critical of myself for my weaknesses or mistakes.

  2 I blame myself all the time for my faults.

  3 I blame myself for everything bad that happens.

9.0 I don't have any thoughts of killing myself.

  1 I have thoughts of killing myself, but I would not carry them out.

  2 I would like to kill myself.

  3 I would kill myself if I had the chance.

10.0 I don't cry any more than usual.

  1 I cry more now than I used to.

  2 I cry all the time now.

  3 I used to be able to cry, but now I can't cry even though I want to.

11.0 I am no more irritated now than I ever am.

   1 I get annoyed or irritated more easily than I used to.

   2 I feel irritated all the time now.

   3 I don't get irritated at all by the things that used to irritate me.

12.0 I have not lost interest in other people.

   1 I am less interested in other people than I used to be.

   2 I have lost most of my interest in other people.

   3 I have lost all of my interest in other people.

13.0 I make decisions as well as I ever could.

   1 I put off making decisions more than I used to.

   2 I have greater difficulty in making decisions than before.

   3 I can't make decisions at all anymore.

14.0 I don't feel I look any worse than I used to.

   1 I am worried that I am looking old or unattractive.

   2 I feel that there are permanent changes in my appearance that make me look unattractive.

   3 I believe that I look ugly.

15.0 I can work about as well as before.

   1 It takes extra effort to get started doing something.

   2 I have to push myself very hard to do anything.

   3 I can't do any work at all.

16.0 I can sleep as well as usual.

   1 I don't sleep as well as I used to.

   2 I wake up 2–3 hours earlier than usual and find it hard to get back to sleep.

3 I wake up several hours earlier than I used to and cannot get back to sleep.

17.0 I don't get more tired than usual.

1 I get tired more easily than I used to.

2 I get tired from doing almost anything.

3 I am too tired to do anything.

18.0 My appetite is no worse than usual.

1 My appetite is not as good as it used to be.

2 My appetite is much worse now.

3 I have no appetite at all anymore.

19.0 I haven't lost much weight, if any, lately.

1 I have lost more than 5 pounds.

2 I have lost more than 10 pounds.

3 I have lost more than 15 pounds.

20.0 I am no more worried about my health than usual.

1 I am worried about physical problems such as aches and pains, or upset stomach, or constipation.

2 I am very worried about physical problems and it's hard to think about anything else.

3 I am so worried about my physical problems that I cannot think about anything else.

21.0 I have not noticed any recent change in my interest in sex.

1 I am less interested in sex than I used to be.

2 I am much less interested in sex now.

3 I have lost interest in sex completely.

The BDI is scored by adding the numbers of the separate items selected. Do not score weight lost on purpose (item 19). A score of 0–9 would be considered in the normal range, 10–15 would suggest mild depression, 16-23 would be consistent with moderate depression, and a score of 24 or more suggests marked depression.

We feel anyone who scores between 10 and 23 should repeat the BDI in two weeks. If the score is still between 10 and 23, and particularly if it has risen, a doctor should be consulted for an evaluation. If the score is greater than 23, a prompt evaluation is certainly indicated. If the score is less than 10 but other indications of depression exist, evaluation is also wise." (The BDI and scoring instructions are reprinted from John W. Griest and James W. Jefferson's book, *Depression and Its Treatment,* pp. 22–26, by permission of the publisher, American Psychiatric Press, Inc., Washington, D.C., published in 1985.)

numb you out) or you don't have a competent doctor who understands how to treat depression (psychiatrists, who are also MDs, are trained in this) and a competent therapist who believes that your past affects your future and who encourages you to look at all the unresolved pain inside, switch to another doctor and therapist right now. Thousands of people are successfully treated for depression every day. There is no need to suffer.

For those of you who are contemplating suicide, you're not going to like it when I tell you this . . . but you are not free from depression just because you leave your physical body. That depression is deep in your soul. It needs to heal, but death will not heal it. The depression will follow you wherever you go. Death is not the answer to depression. It is a problem with known solutions that are sometimes surprisingly simple.

Beth came to me once a week for several months to get healings for her depression. Each time, I would lay my hands on her, channeling a healing to release whatever issues were inside her body. Each week a different issue would come up: painful memories of her mother; hurt and disappointment in her marital relationship; negative beliefs that said she was unlovable, unworthy, bad, a burden, incapable, inferior, inadequate, unwanted, worthless. Beth was seeing me, in addition to a therapist and a chiropractor. She had suffered from depression most of her life and finally got tired of it, deciding that instead of being a victim, she would do whatever she could to heal it. She made daily progress in her healing, taking charge of her life and no longer allowing depression to stop her from going forward.

In a psychic reading, my spirit guide John gave her this prayer to say each day to help with the healing:

> Don't let me stay stuck in my negativity, in my anger. Push me past the place I am now. Push me. Push me to go deeper in my relationship with God and myself. Push me. Help me change my patterns . . . to see myself as a different person . . . a child of God who is capable of anything. Help me take the blinders off my eyes and see myself clearly. Thank you.

If you are feeling stuck, I suggest that you say this prayer every day for thirty days. Hopefully, you will soon be able to make your depression a thing of the past.

Depression and the Holidays

Holidays can be wonderful, bringing family and friends together. People express love and joy for each other. But holidays can also be depressing. They can remind us of the unhealed separation and hurt in our lives.

Holidays evoke feelings of all kinds. For instance, there are usually two very distinct reactions to Christmas: people are either totally into it or they hate it. Some people don't react to it one way or another. The same is true to a lesser or greater degree with all the holidays: Hanukkah, Thanksgiving, New Year's Eve, Valentine's Day, Easter, as well as the one special day that is not considered a legal holiday but is, I believe a very important day—your birthday!

What were the messages in your family about the holidays? Were they positive or negative? Do the holidays make you happy? Sad? Lonely? Miserable? Uptight? Anxious? It is often said that the holidays are the loneliest time of the year for thousands and thousands of people.

Whatever memories or feelings you come up with, you can make a change, starting now, about how you will experience all future holidays and birthdays. Let yourself feel *everything* that comes up for you concerning holidays, and feel free to write and talk about these feelings. You may think your feelings may be trite or unimportant, but in my healing practice I see many people every year who are deeply affected by the holidays.

Remember, you can get free from all the old garbage. Do the recommended exercise at the end of this chapter. You don't have to be victimized by the holidays!

Journal Work

Exercise 1

Areas of Stress

Divide a page in your journal into two columns of approximately equal sizes. Label the left column "My Stresses," the right one "Where I Hold the Stress."

Think about areas of your life where you are feeling particularly stressed: money, people, job, school, children, parents, brothers or sisters, illness, weather, car trouble, commute problems, and the like. Write down everything that causes you to feel stressed. As you are writing, notice how your body is feeling. Are any aches and pains rearing their little heads? Are you becoming aware of a pain that has been there for quite a while? Write down whatever awareness you are having about your body.

Exercise 2

Evaluate Your Depression Level

If you feel you may be suffering from depression, or have occasionally gone through bouts of depression in the past, use the Beck Depression Inventory to evaluate yourself. If you find that you score between 10 and 23, repeat the inventory in two weeks. If your score is still within that range or is even higher, consult with a physician, preferably a psychiatrist who is skilled in the treatment of depression. Remember, depression is one of the most common illnesses seen by doctors, and there are effective treatment programs that make it completely unnecessary for you to suffer any longer.

Exercise 3

Holiday Word Association

Read over the following list very slowly. When you come across a word that brings up strong feelings of any kind, record in your journal what that word is and what you are feeling. Here is the list:

Thanksgiving

Hanukkah

Presents

Santa Claus

Money

Children

Christmas tree

Hanukkah bush

Friends

Receiving cards

Traffic/parking

Recent painful holidays

Christmas

Shopping

Cookies/candy/holiday treats

Snow

Parties

Mom/Dad

Family gatherings

Traveling

Sending cards

Department stores

Expectations you have of others

Exercise 4

The Way I'd Like It to Be

Ask yourself how you would like holidays and birthdays to be. What changes would you like to make to ensure that future holidays or birthdays are less stressful? Note these changes in your journal.

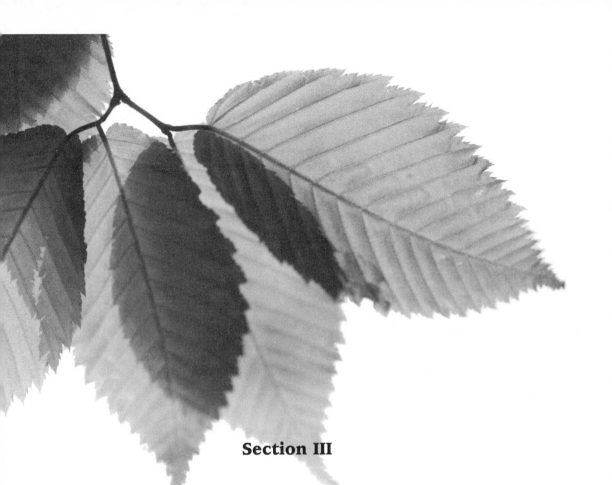

Section III

Gender and Healing

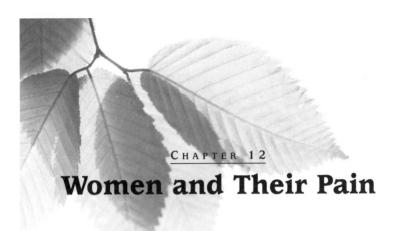

CHAPTER 12

Women and Their Pain

*S**uddenly I find myself churning inside like a trou-
bled sea.*

—Natalie Rogers

Sandra, a woman in her early forties who was suffering from extreme fatigue, came to me recently for a healing. She was married and had a two-year-old child, and she was a supervisor in a large corporation. Although Sandra loved her job, her husband, and her child, her life was extremely hectic, and she was having trouble doing all that was expected of her. She had a difficult time asking anyone, including her husband, for help. With a full-time job and primary responsibility for raising her child, Sandra still tried to be attractive at the end of the day. Yet Sandra felt guilty when she complained about her life because it was all "really very nice."

When I channeled healing energy to her, Sandra would cry and cry. Her body felt very sad about all that was expected of her each day. Her body really wanted a break!

Her medical doctors finally discovered that she had mononucleosis and told her that she was not to work for quite some time. I believe that her illness was her body's only way of getting her to slow down and make some changes in her life. She continued to come to me for healings, and it became increasingly obvious that she needed to change some of her attitudes and beliefs about herself and what was expected of her.

Gradually, Sandra learned to delegate some of her responsibilities. She learned to say no when she felt stretched to the limit. She accepted that she had limitations, which was really difficult for her to do. She looked at her physical problem in a holistic way. What had caused her to get sick? What did it mean mentally, emotionally, and spiritually, as well as physically? She made some tremendous changes because she was open to them and to the necessary healing. As a result, Sandra healed quickly.

What It Means to Be a Woman

Let's look at what being a woman means to you. First of all, do you like being a woman? Do you like the way your life is? In general, are you happy with your role as a woman?

Are you a mother? Do you have a full-time job? Do you go to school? Are you in a relationship? Do you care for your parents or members of your family other than your children? Do you have a lot of responsibility? Do you ask for help when you need it? Are you the person you always wanted to be, or are you living the way others would like you to live?

In the past few years I find myself doing healings for more and more women caught up in "superwoman" roles. I can see what all of the stress is doing to their bodies, especially when it is coupled with unresolved issues and the emotions surrounding them.

Many women are angry about their treatment by society in general and by co-workers, family members, and even other women. I've seen women with mononucleosis, lupus, chronic fatigue syndrome, fibromyalgia, asthma, and clinical depression. Every one of them has a very difficult schedule, juggling school, children, a full-time career, a relationship, or all of the above. They all knew before getting sick that they should slow down, make changes in their lives, delegate some of their responsibilities. But they just kept pushing themselves until they became physically sick.

Over the past few years I have also seen many women who are having trouble getting pregnant. One woman in her thirties was a very busy professional. She was also in school finishing her postgraduate studies. She and her new husband had just purchased a home, a fixer-upper, and were trying to get pregnant but with no luck.

I remember psychically looking inside her body, trying to get some information that would help with her inability to conceive. Her body said to me:

> No way! I will not get pregnant. I'm already exhausted. I can only handle so much and right now I'm stressed to the limit with tight schedules and heavy demands on me. Tell her I will get pregnant only when there is a change in our lifestyle and I'm not expected to do so much all the time.

Her body also shared its fear concerning her husband's ambivalence about being a parent. It was afraid she was going to have to do all the parenting herself. Her body said there was a great deal to be figured out and changed before it would open itself up to a baby.

It is my belief that many of the health challenges women are having today are directly related to their role as women. It's very difficult for many women to say no, to put themselves at the top of their own priority lists. It's difficult for them to delegate responsibilities to others or to accept their own limitations. It is difficult for them to receive rather than always give.

For this reason it is more important than ever to take a very close look at our expectations for ourselves, the expectations of others, and how these expectations may be causing us some physical problems.

Women and Sexuality

Perhaps one of the most difficult areas for women to resolve and to integrate into their lives in a healthy way is their sexuality. I have done several healings over the years for women who are struggling with being sexual. Usually these issues manifest themselves physically through the following:

ovulation problems

PMS (premenstrual
  syndrome)

difficult menstrual periods

fibroid cysts in the breasts

vaginal infections

ovarian and uterine cysts

fibroid tumors

herpes

cancer

difficult menopause

Anna, a twenty-five-year-old art student, came to me for an intense two-and-a-half-hour healing. She wanted to be free of her negative feelings around sexuality. When I psychically looked at Anna's body, her negative attitudes, beliefs, and feelings were in her breasts. I saw images of past lives when she had bound up her breasts to hide them. There were feelings of shame around being a woman. She said that in this life she would often wear a very restricting bra to make her look smaller. She was trying to hide her femaleness.

John, my spirit guide, said that her negative attitudes and beliefs around her sexuality, her femaleness, her wants and desires as a woman, and her sexual needs were all issues she came into this lifetime to heal. Anna cried a lot during our sessions. I could feel the energy healing past-life pain. Many past-life images came to her as I channeled the energy.

It was an incredible healing! Anna told me that she was convinced that the healings, along with working on her emotional issues with her therapist, had saved her from developing breast cancer. She said that ever since her breasts began to develop, she could feel an inner tenseness about them. It was as if she wished that they weren't there.

I have also seen numerous women struggle with their lack of sexual desires. One such woman was Maria, a fifty-two-year-old woman who came in for healings of a recurring bladder infection. Maria told me that her husband really got on her nerves. She always felt angry with him. She didn't want to have sex with him, but didn't want to appear frigid either. So her body created a monthly bladder problem. This condition had continued for more than a year. The payoff was that her husband not only didn't ask her to have sex but was nice to her each time that she got another infection.

For Maria's healings to be complete, she had to address the issues she had with her husband by talking them out. I told her that if her bladder healed without resolving these issues, their emotional root would manifest in some other physical way. But Maria chose to keep the bladder issues rather than to examine her issues with her husband. She simply refused to go to the root of her problem.

I had another client, a flight attendant named Abby, who felt extremely bitter toward her ex-husband. They had met on a flight, and at first she had been drawn to his commanding personality. But shortly after they were married, he began wanting to have a lot of kinky sex, and intercourse with him, which she had previously enjoyed, began to disgust her. She felt that it was her duty to have sex with him, so she never said no. Eventually, she was able to leave him.

After they had been divorced for a few months, Abby began suffering from a lot of pain inside her vagina. It was very red and swollen, and constantly itched.

John told me that Abby was just as angry at herself for not saying no as she was toward her ex-husband for wanting kinky sex. She needed to forgive both of them. Abby's healing process was long and painful. She cried on and off for weeks, which was very necessary. As we were healing layers of memories, other memories from her childhood surfaced. She had blocked out sexual abuse by her grandfather. This also needed to be healed.

Emotional Roots

As a woman, it is easy for me to identify with others' struggles around their sexuality. I believe that the sexual abuse I experienced as a child, as well as the double messages I got about being female, were the emotional roots of most of my female problems. Like many of the women I have seen over the years with the same or similar issues, I didn't want to be sexual, so my body created problems to use as an excuse. I have also seen women who have guilt about enjoying themselves sexually or who are not married and feel guilty about having sex. Their bodies created vaginal problems as a form of self-punishment.

Looking at issues around sex can really be tough. I had been in therapy on and off for years, had talked about my confusion around sex, had talked about the sexual abuse. But until I was in my thirties I never really felt my anger or rage or sadness around these experiences. When I was twenty-nine, I went into surgically induced menopause after having a total hysterectomy. My ovaries, my fallopian tubes, my uterus, and my cervix were covered with benign tumors.

Today, I know that my reproductive organs had stored all of my feelings of rage, anger, sadness, hopelessness, resentment, and self-pity around being a woman. These unresolved feelings turned into benign tumors. I think my body was saying, "Echo, I can't or don't want to be a dumping ground for all of your negative feelings anymore."

Shortly after the hysterectomy, I went into a severe depression and suffered from several physical and emotional symptoms, which I later realized was menopause: hot flashes, nervousness, paranoia, anxiety, forgetfulness, and insomnia. Until I was put on the correct dosage of hormone replacement, every day was a nightmare. This actually turned out to be a blessing in disguise because I went back into therapy and really began looking at all of my issues around my sexuality and being a woman.

Most women I have known or done healings for have found it difficult to look at their feelings about being a woman. Are you having any recurring female problems, that is, trouble with any area of your body that identifies you as a woman or that has anything to do with your sexuality? Can you identify your feelings about being sexual? Perhaps going back to chapter 7 will help you identify them. You'll have an opportunity to do more work on this topic in the journal work section at the end of this chapter.

Wakeup Call

You deserve a happy, productive, stress-free, joy-filled life— not because of how hard you work or how good you look. You deserve it just because you are you. It is your birthright.

If you are a woman and don't like it, if you are having difficulty with your role as a woman, or if you are having difficulty with your sexuality, you have suffered long enough. It's time to start healing. It's time to get free from this pain. The process will probably not be any more painful than the pain with which you already live. And once you have gone through it, you'll be free of it. The pain will end.

My belief is that, as women, we are fortunate. We can find ways to have it all, all meaning anything we want—career, family, creativity, education, our own income, our own spirituality, rewarding friendships, fulfilling relationships. Society's attitude, in general, is changing toward women. More and more doors open for us each day.

But we can't have it all if we don't feel good.

Journal Work

Exercise 1

Your Feelings about Being a Woman

In your journal, write down your feelings about being a woman. It can be most helpful to go back to the list in chapter 7. Write down what you feel about women in general and about your own role as a woman. What expectations do you have as a woman? Write down everything that comes to mind, allowing yourself to free-associate as you do.

Exercise 2

Your Sexuality

Part A

Look at your feelings around your sexuality. Are you sexually active? How do you feel about it? Are you not sexually active? How do you feel about that?

Record your responses in your journal.

Part B

Ask yourself if there are any parts of your body that are feeling fearful or tense right now. Write those down and describe what you are experiencing.

Part C

Are there any questions you are hoping I won't ask? What are they and why are you hoping I won't ask?

Exercise 3

Connecting Feelings to Physical Problems

Do you see any connection between your attitudes and beliefs about being a woman, your sexuality, and any physical problems you may be having? Please write these down in your journal.

Exercise 4

Inner-Child Work

Put your pencil or pen in your nondominant hand and ask your inner child how it feels about being female. Don't edit its thoughts and feelings. Let it be as expressive as possible.

Now ask it to write how it feels about sex. Ask it if it has any memories of being hurt by someone sexually.

Remember, its answers will be different from yours. Its words or pictures may be different from the ones you would use, but that doesn't matter. Just let it express itself so that you can get to the bottom of any memories that might be hiding inside.

Exercise 5

The Adult You

Once I became honest with myself and my therapist about the rage I felt, and began releasing the negative and hurtful feelings I had around being sexual, I began to heal. I began to see the positive aspects of being a woman. We are beautiful, creative, spontaneous, passionate, loving, nurturing, playful, delightful human beings.

Part A

Write down in your journal your positive feelings and beliefs about being a woman. If you don't presently have any, move on to part B.

Part B

Write down what you hope you will one day feel about being a woman.

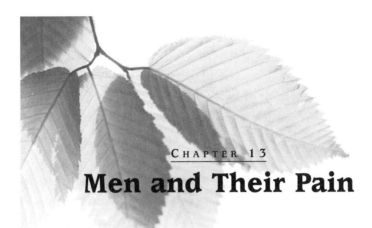

CHAPTER 13

Men and Their Pain

*W*hen a man's self is hidden from everybody else
*. . . it seems also to become much hidden even
from himself, and it permits disease and death
to gnaw into his substance without his clear
knowledge.*

—Sidney Jourard

As a spiritual healer, I worry about men and their health. I see
them as the real victims in a society that discourages them from
expressing their emotions. I watch the boys playing in my neigh-
borhood, and I have noticed that at a very early age they ridicule
each other if they show any signs of pain, such as crying, when
they are hurt. I worry about the long-term effect this will have on
their health.

When I psychically look inside men to see what's going on, I
find that their bodies aren't as easy to read as are the bodies of
women. I believe this is because men aren't given permission to
express their feelings, and begin storing their pain at a very early

age. Sometimes I see images of painful experiences inside them. But the men are usually so detached from their emotional memories and pain that they can't connect with the images I see.

The Hazards of Being Male by Dr. Herb Goldberg was a difficult book for me to read because it really made me aware of the pain men experience. In a chapter titled "Impossible Binds," the author says:

> The male in our culture finds himself in countless "damned if you do, damned if you don't" no-win binds. He is constantly being affected by gross inconsistencies— between what he had been taught was "masculine" behavior as a boy and what is expected of him as an adult; between inner needs and social pressures; and between contradictory expectations in the many roles he has to play. He is psychologically fragmented by these many contradictory demands.

Goldberg goes on to say that for survival's sake, most men are literally forced into being emotionally detached and out of touch with feelings of any kind. He states:

> The traditional male façade—cool, detached, controlled, guarded, and disengaged—is a protective mechanism that allows him to respond simply to external cues or inputs, like a programmed computer, rather than having to wrestle with constant conflict and ambiguity. The first step in coping with this phenomenon is open recognition and acknowledgment of these binds. (p. 86)

Goldberg describes many different binds that affect men's lives. One of the most devastating, in terms of our present discussion, is what he calls the "feeling bind." He points out that throughout life the male who expresses his feelings openly, or who "readily cries, screams, behaves sensually, etc.," learns that he may be looked upon as neurotic or unstable. By controlling his feelings, as he is expected to do, he "will inevitably become guarded, hidden, and emotionally unknown to himself and others and viewed as 'cold' and even hostile." Either way the man ends up losing. If he lets it all hang out, he is viewed as immature or "unmanly," lacking self-control. But if he holds in his emotions he is accused of being secretive, unemotional, and "overly self-controlled."

Goldberg goes on to say that a man can be released from impossible binds by reclaiming the deep feelings that lie hidden behind his defenses, recognizing and accepting them as part of himself. He may see them as a threatening part of himself, but at least then he can be in a position to choose whether or not he is going to risk being true to the real self behind his defenses. Goldberg points out:

> Undoubtedly, the re-owning of the real self will precipitate a crisis in the lives of all men who have allowed themselves to be bound up in these annihilating conflicts. It may therefore be necessary to acknowledge the need for help with these struggles and to seek it from a competent therapist. (p. 97)

Mixed Messages

If you are a man, mixed messages may be causing you many physical problems, as well as emotional ones.

Men receive so many mixed messages. They are told to get their anger out, yet are reminded not to lose their tempers. They are told they need to express their feelings more, yet we give them another message that says, "Don't be too emotional because that is a sign of weakness." We want them to be more sensitive. More romantic. More sentimental. On the other hand, we say, "Go off to war and protect us. Kill whomever you have to, just don't come back and tell us about it. Come back and be the loving, sensitive, trusting, romantic guy you were before you left."

Most men have learned to deny their feelings, wants, desires, needs, and physical pain. They feel they are supposed to strive harder, compete, and yet be nice guys. They don't know how to reach out to friends because they are taught at an early age to compete with others. When they do socialize, the conversations are not deep and elaborate but tend to be superficial. Men learn to avoid topics that would make them appear needy. As Goldberg points out, a man's inner life is filled with lessons that put him in emotional double-binds or impossible-binds and leave him lonely and in despair.

Doug, a thirty-year-old man suffering from diabetes, came to me for healings for more than five years. Almost immediately, I saw images inside his pancreas of a great deal of shame around his leaving the Seventh-Day Adventist Church in which he had been raised. I asked him about this, and here is what he told me:

> The impact of joining the SDA Church saturated every facet of my life. Suddenly, we were very active churchgoers. We went to church at least four to five times per week; we studied daily Sabbath school lessons; we became vegetarians; and we were active in church missions and associated primarily with church members. There were shames for not being more holy, and we were entreated to be more obedient or we would go to Hell. There was immense guilt for breaking any of the rules.

Doug went on to tell me that when he turned twenty-five, he decided to leave the church against his family's wishes. Within weeks, he came down with diabetes.

During each of our healing sessions, Doug worked on several issues as they slowly surfaced, one by one. First, there were the layers and layers of shame about his decision to go against the family and the church. Doug also struggled with his relationship with God, because for a long time he truly believed God had given him the disease of diabetes as punishment. His issues around sexuality and people-pleasing also surfaced. Doug was always being "Mr. Nice Guy," saying yes to everyone so as not to rock the boat or cause anyone to get upset. He had to learn that it was okay to do and be what felt right for him in spite of what any others wanted or needed him to do.

The healings brought up many memories of past pain, and Doug eventually sought the help of a therapist who helped him heal emotionally. It was fascinating to watch the process of a wonderful combination of spiritual and emotional healing.

Roles and Expectations

I see so many men struggle for their freedom from the roles and expectations society has placed on them. Many men choose to go along with what's expected of them rather than go through the hassle of challenging the status quo. They avoid making major changes because it seems easier that way. But again, consider the price for this in terms of their health!

In my opinion, many of the heart attacks men suffer are broken hearts—literally the injured hearts of people who never lived the way they wanted to. They got caught up in doing what was expected of them.

No doubt the most challenging and harmful expectation we place on men is sending them off to war, to "serve their country." I've seen several men who served in the armed forces; one client comes to mind. He was a man in his early forties with bad knees and chronic back, neck, and shoulder problems. When I looked inside, I saw memories of Vietnam: hate, rage, sadness that he had to go, and for all that he saw and had to do. Resentment for losing four years of his youth. I asked him if he cried or yelled out his feelings. He replied, "What good would it do?"

> In the movie *Prince of Tides* the psychiatrist asks the brother of his patient, "Did you ever cry over your brother's death?"
> "What good would it do; it wouldn't bring him back," he says.
> The psychiatrist replies, "No, but it might bring you back!"

I see so many men full of old pain, old memories, old injustices done to them. But for some reason or other, they don't want to go inside and get that old baggage out of there. Many don't believe the past can affect them as much as it does. Many struggle with the idea that unresolved issues could be sitting inside their bodies, preferring not to believe that such a thing might be possible.

One saving grace for men is physical activity. Exercise can work a lot of old pain out of the body, but I also believe that if some really serious issues are in there, issues such as sexual, physical, or emotional abuse, they need to be talked out with a competent therapist and dealt with. If not, they will forever affect all current and future relationships with co-workers, significant others, children—and themselves!

Men must learn to listen to the warning signals that their bodies send out when something is wrong. (Women aren't very good at this either.) They must learn not to deny physical or emotional pain because it isn't "manly." They must learn it is okay not to go to work when they don't feel well, and that they won't appear helpless or dependent. Staying in bed because of sickness is the only acceptable way they can pamper themselves—but many won't even do that. Men pride themselves on not missing any time at work, which is another reason they don't pay attention to those early warning signals from their bodies. They have a tendency to want to prove that they can resist, ignore, and overcome signs of illness.

We all—men and women—need to be more sensitive to our bodies, to listen to our dreams and be true to ourselves.

Get rid of the layers of other people's expectations: your mom's, your dad's, your partner's, your children's, your boss's. Peel away those layers of other people's wants, needs, and desires for you. Get down to your own. You are in there somewhere! Please, give yourself a chance to survive the hazards of being male.

Only you can free yourself from the internal pain that is common to most men. Without hurting yourself or anyone else, do whatever you've got to do to begin to heal.

Journal Work

Exercise 1

An Inventory of Fundamental Needs

Go over the following list of questions, answering each one as honestly as possible. As you go along, record in your journal any thoughts, ideas, or feelings that come up.

1. Do you feel your feelings?

2. Do you get nurturing from others?

3. Can you take care of yourself emotionally? Physically?

4. Can you cry? Do you?

5. Do you ask for what you need?

6. Do you know what you need?

7. Do you know and have conversations with the kind of people you would like to?

8. Do you have friendships with other men?

9. Are they satisfying for you?

10. What do you do when you feel sad?

11. Who protects you?

12. Who was or is your hero? Why?

13. What are your burdens?

14. What do you do when you feel angry? Enraged?

15. What do you do when you are physically hurt?

16. Do you ask for help when you need it?

17. What do you do when you make a mistake?

18. How do you feel when you make a mistake?

19. What do you expect from other men, in general?

20. Have you ever lost a family member or close friend? How did you deal with the loss?

21. Are you happy with your sexuality?

22. Are you the kind of sexual partner you want to be?

23. Do you express yourself sexually?

24. Do you allow yourself to express your passion?

25. How do you express your creativity?

26. Do you have a hobby?

27. Do you ever let your imagination flow?

28. Do you have a lot of pride? Where does it show up?

29. What limitations do you feel as far as being a man?

30. When was the last time someone held you? Comforted you?

31. When was the last time someone bought you a present?

32. Do you ever worry about losing control?

33. What do you think would happen if you let go of feelings such as: Sadness? Anger? Frustration? Guilt? Shame?

34. Has your heart ever been broken? What did you do with the feelings you had? What did you do with your feelings of loss?

35. Did you allow yourself to feel the pain, or did you try to replace the feelings of loss with something else?

36. What about your body? Does it look the way you'd like it to?

37. Do you have an image of the way you are supposed to look?

38. How do you express your joy?

39. Do you feel responsible for other people? Who? Why?

40. What regrets do you have?

41. What makes you feel guilty?

42. Do you respect yourself?

43. Do people take you seriously?

44. Do you take yourself seriously?

45. What is weakness to you?

46. What do you do when you watch a sad movie?

47. As a child, what were the messages you received from adult males in your life about being a man?

48. As a child, what were the messages you received from adult women in your life about being a man? What were their expectations?

49. What is it like for you to be a man?

50. What would you like to change about yourself or your life?

Notice that there are no "right" or "wrong" answers here. These are questions that each person will answer in his own way.

Exercise 2

The Little Boy Within

With your nondominant hand, ask your little boy inside what it's been like for him to be a boy. Then ask him to write down what it has been like for him to be a man.

Exercise 3

War Experiences

One of the most difficult experiences a person can face is having to go to war. While many men consider it a man's duty to "serve his country" in this way, it is nevertheless inevitable that they will have strong feelings about it after they get out. If you are a veteran of any armed conflict, take this opportunity to get in touch with what the experience meant for you.

Part A

Record in your journal any memories or feelings that come up for you around serving your country in an armed conflict.

Part B

If you did not serve in an armed conflict, you may still have feelings about not serving. Write them down in your journal.

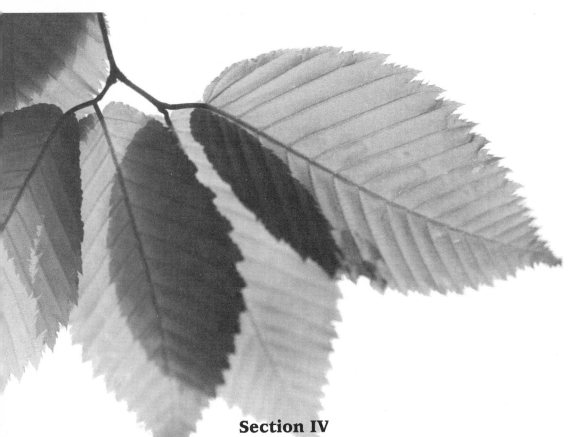

Section IV

Pathways to Healing

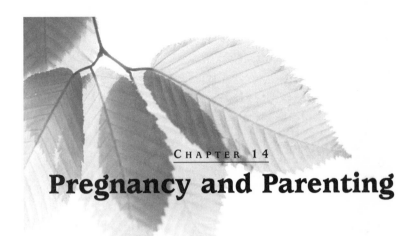

CHAPTER 14

Pregnancy and Parenting

*S*ome *parents judge themselves quite harshly. . . .*
We all wish we were able to live our ideals . . . yet
it seems so important to be compassionate toward
the person we were at that time, to be under-
standing and forgiving.

—Michael Gabriel

In this section, we'll explore the pathways to healing, visiting those areas of our lives where our deepest fears and conflicts tend to play themselves out. Here's where the hot buttons get pushed, where we summon defense strategies, worn-out excuses, lies, and deceptions, hurting those we love and hurting ourselves in an effort to hang on to our negative beliefs. These are also the life experiences that promote healing. Difficult as it is, we can let go of our destructive patterns or we can continue to fight the same old battles about the same old things in the same old ways. The choice is ours.

We begin with pregnancy and parenting, a subject that should be light, romantic, and joyful. The movies always seem to make it so. Parents-to-be are usually very much in love. The woman finds a cute, clever way to tell the man how much she loves the fact that they are going to have a baby. They ride off into the sunset, have the perfect baby, and all live happily (and perfectly) ever after.

Unfortunately, in many cases, getting pregnant can be a very painful experience emotionally: teenage pregnancy, pregnancy through rape, pregnancy out of wedlock, unplanned pregnancy. The pregnancy can prematurely end in a miscarriage or be terminated by abortion. There's the pain of giving birth to a stillborn child or giving birth to a child who is considered "less than perfect," which means that there is a physical deformity or a mental disorder. Then there are the parents who go through the pain of Sudden Infant Death Syndrome (SIDS). A pregnancy may end in adoption or placing the child in a foster home. At the opposite end of the spectrum there is the pain of not being able to get pregnant.

Even under the best of circumstances, most people do not think very far ahead when they get pregnant. Many are ill-equipped to be parents and are unable to face the challenges that may lie ahead. What if that precious infant does not become the son or daughter they always wanted? What if the child turns out to be a disappointment or an embarrassment?

I have seen in my own case, and in those of many of my clients, how conflicts around pregnancy, children, and parenting that stem from unresolved issues can create some real health problems physically, mentally, and emotionally. But this "combat zone" is also a healing battleground—a place where the challenges that present themselves are also an opportunity.

Unplanned Pregnancy

When I was nineteen years old, I found out that I was pregnant. I had not used any means of contraception for two reasons: first, the doctor had told me that because of my poor history of ovulating I wouldn't be able to get pregnant without medical help; second, I felt guilty about having sex before marriage. Using birth control was an admission that I was no longer what I was supposed to be—a virgin.

My boyfriend, my parents, and I weighed the pros and cons of what I should do about the pregnancy. Abortion didn't feel right to me, and neither did marriage. We were so young. Our relationship wasn't the healthiest. I was terrified of being a mother and a wife.

We decided that I would go to California, stay with friends of our families, have the baby, put it up for adoption, and then come back to Minnesota. We were embarrassed to tell anyone the truth, so we told friends that I was transferring to college in Palo Alto. In 1968, being pregnant and not married was a pretty shameful thing. In addition, being in California on my own was difficult because I had never been away from home prior to this. I earned money by babysitting. I wore a ring from Woolworth's and told everyone my husband was in Vietnam.

As tough as it was, I loved being pregnant, having the feeling of life inside me. I talked to my baby all of the time, holding my stomach as if I were holding him. I explained to him that I loved him more than anything and didn't want to give him up, but felt as if I should. I was so afraid that he would not feel loved. I spent many hours crying about the way it was all going to turn out. Even though I knew he was going to a good family, I was always trying to think of a way to keep him for myself. If there really was a God, I couldn't understand why a woman would have to give up her baby.

My son was born on November 20, 1968. Three days later, I returned to Minnesota, forty pounds heavier than when I had left. I had gained so much weight because I ate all of the time. I didn't know how to deal with all of my feelings around the pregnancy. Everyone thought that I was coming back from school, so no one could understand why I seemed so depressed. I had terrible post-partum blues that lasted for weeks.

I stayed in my room, not ever wanting to come out. I never wanted to see another man as long as I lived; I never wanted to have sex again either. However, in my state of confusion I wanted at the same time to get my baby back and marry his father. I didn't know what was right anymore. I felt miserable and moped around for about three months. Finally, my father insisted that I get a job or go back to college. He also bought me a health club membership.

I got a job as a night manager at a pancake house. I went on a diet and worked out at the club but, unfortunately, I didn't do anything about my emotional state. So many of us think that if we just have a good job and look good on the outside, any emotional problems on the inside will go away. I did everything I could to improve myself on the outside and began my search for Mr. Right. I became almost obsessed with getting married and replacing my baby.

I am telling you this story because I know that I am not the only one who has gone through this experience. The effects of this pregnancy lasted for more than twenty years. Every year after my son was born, from the beginning of October (the original estimated due date) until the 20th of November (the delivery date), I would go into a state of deep depression. I would feel a very heavy sense of loss. Mentally, I would become very preoccupied, almost as if I were someplace else, but I could not make out what was happening to me. My family and close friends noticed my behavior. Every year I would tell myself that I wasn't going to go through it again and, just like clockwork, the first week in October I would slowly start to slip into a depression. I would go to therapy early in the fall to ward it off before it began, but there seemed to be no way to control it.

I told the story over and over again, but never really got into my feelings of shame, humiliation, fear, anger, resentment, and guilt. I listed the facts—first this happened, then that happened—but I didn't talk about how I humiliated I had felt when people asked me about my husband or wanted to plan a baby shower for me. I felt so ashamed of myself when I ducked out of town immediately after leaving the hospital. I knew it was my way of avoiding telling anyone the truth.

I wouldn't have to talk about how I had disappointed my parents, or how I was fearful that my brother would no longer like me or would think I was a slut. I wouldn't have to mention the shame I felt when the hospital put me in a room away from the other mothers to avoid upsetting them. I wouldn't have to admit to the incredible amount of pain I felt each time I sat outside the nursery window staring at my baby, knowing I would never touch him or be with him. Or the terrible sadness I felt when I could feel a child inside me—my child—which I was going to give away. The truth was no matter how many times people had told me that it was such an unselfish and loving thing to put my child up for adoption, it didn't relieve that deep sense of sorrow.

All of those feelings sat in my body for years. The tapes in my body played over and over again: "I am bad. I am an embarrassment to others. I am messed up. I am no good. I can't do anything right. I am a failure. I hurt other people. I am a disgrace."

I told therapist after therapist that I was a bad person. I told all the stories in great detail so they would understand why I felt the way I did, but it didn't seem to relieve the beliefs or the feelings I had. I wanted to stay away from the feelings because they were too painful to experience again. I believe today that the reason I stayed stuck for so long was because I stayed in my head and talked about the facts of my pregnancy rather than the feelings associated with my pregnancy.

When I finally started to feel my feelings about my pregnancy and the loss of my child, sharing them with my therapist, I began to heal. My therapist suggested that I really grieve my loss. At first, I responded that I had cried every year over my loss. She told me that even though I had cried, I had never really let my son go and so had never really grieved my loss. I cried off and on for the next week about this. I had to give myself permission just to cry, cry, cry . . . to get the sadness out of my body.

Healing the Pain of Pregnancy

I had a client named Rebecca who still held her resentments in her uterus as the result of a pregnancy she had twenty-three years earlier!

Rebecca's husband Dan had not wanted a baby and thought his wife felt the same. When she became pregnant, he felt betrayed and did nothing to support her. He refused to participate in child-birth classes, and when she was in labor, he chose to go fishing.

For twenty-three years Rebecca held on to those resentments, and finally they grew into several benign tumors in her uterus. She told me that she never shared with her husband how deeply hurt she was because she didn't want to upset him.

Do you have any negative issues relating to a pregnancy or pregnancies, either in the past or at the present time? Review this list of questions and see whether any pertain to you:

1. Was your pregnancy difficult and/or you had no support?

2. When you first found out you were pregnant, were you anxious or fearful?

3. Did you choose to have an abortion? Have you grieved that loss?

4. Do you have feelings of shame or anger or guilt about having had an abortion? Have you ever dealt with those feelings?

5. Perhaps, at the time of an abortion you thought: "I don't want to think about it. I just want to do it and get on with my life." How have those stored feelings affected you over time?

6. Were you single when you found out that you were pregnant? Did you go through the pregnancy alone?

7. If you were single, what happened to the child's other parent? What were people's attitudes toward you? What was your attitude toward yourself? Did you feel anger, sadness, shame, guilt, remorse, or hatred? All of these things?

8. Did you go through a pregnancy that ended painfully, such as an adoption or a stillbirth?

9. After your child's entrance into the world, did you discover that she was physically or mentally impaired? Have you wondered what you could have done differently? Or you have shut down your heart because you don't want to feel pain, disappointment, anger, hurt, or fear?

10. Have you been unable to get pregnant? If your partner is the one with the problems, do you feel resentment toward her?

If any of these questions are too painful for you to think about, it means that the pain is still inside, locked in.

Parenting

Parenting is another area of our lives that has the potential to become a source of healing, if we can overcome the pain and conflict surrounding choices made or choices that were forced upon us. Parenting is also a legacy from our own parents, and how we were raised will dictate much of the emotional pain we carry and subsequently bring into the lives of our own children.

The circumstances of how we became a parent may have a lot to do with how we feel about this role. See if any of the following questions pertain to you:

1. Are you a parent by choice?

2. Did you have different plans, goals, or dreams for yourself? Do you have resentments toward the child or your partner?

3. Are you one of the millions of people who are raising your child or children single-handedly?

4. If you are a single parent, how are you coping with this role? Do you ever feel cheated? Resentful? Angry, alone, ashamed, judged, overwhelmed, afraid, or remorseful? Is it a hardship financially?

5. If you are raising your child alone, do you have negative feelings toward the child's other parent?

Again, if any of these questions resonate with you or are too painful for you to think about, it is likely that the pain is still stored somewhere in your body.

During healings with single mothers, I have seen many negative feelings toward the child's father or the child itself residing in the pelvic area where they are now causing or will eventually cause pain or illness.

I have also had male clients who are raising their children alone. Some feel like victims of circumstances. Sadly, they either take their feelings out on their children or hold them inside. My healings on these men reveal a lot of anger inside their bodies, especially in the back, neck, and shoulders.

Older Children

Let's move beyond pregnancy to your child as she is growing or has grown up. If you have resentment toward your child, these feelings are going to physically hurt you. You have got to get these feelings out of your body. Here are more questions to answer or think about:

1. Is your child the one that you always wanted?

2. Did your child turn out to be a disappointment or an embarrassment?

3. Is your child now a burden on you emotionally or physically?

4. Do you feel jealousy or hatred toward your child?

5. Do you feel rage, frustration, disappointment, hurt, sadness, remorse, guilt, or perhaps even envy that your child has been able to do things in life that you haven't been able to do in yours?

Whatever your feelings about parenting your child, if the outcome hasn't been what you wanted or dreamed about, you can heal from the experience. As you do the exercises in this chapter and elsewhere in this book, be patient with yourself and your body. If tears come, don't hold them back. If you feel angry, yell at the whole crummy, painful situation and tell it how you feel. Beat some pillows if you need to. Just remember not to hurt yourself or your child in this releasing process. There has already been enough hurt for this lifetime.

Journal Work

Exercise 1

Touching Your Feelings

Put your hands on your abdomen and close your eyes. Allow your thoughts to wander back to the time when you were pregnant. Experience any emotions that are stirring up. If you were single and pregnant, or if you were forced to terminate a pregnancy—if you faced parenting alone or put your child up for adoption—whatever choices you made or were forced to make, let your feelings about these choices emerge. As feelings, memories, and awarenesses come to the surface, let them flow. If tears come, let them out. If you feel angry, yell what you are feeling out loud. Take time to fully experience all of your feelings. Then, when you feel ready, record this experience in your healing journal.

Exercise 2

Broken Dreams

Did your pregnancy change your expectations about the way you thought your life would turn out? If you had different plans, goals, or dreams for yourself, do you feel any resentment toward your child, your partner, or perhaps even yourself? Do you feel angry or remorseful about the way your life is turning out? If you were raised a religious person, has this affected your relationship with God? Do you ever feel that God did this to you?

Let yourself experience any feelings that come up. Let yourself recall memories of what you had planned or dreamed for your life. Record the memories and feelings that come up in your journal.

Exercise 3

The Adoption/Foster Home Dilemma

Over the past forty years I've done readings for many people who were adopted and have never met one that didn't want to know why. As part of your healing process, I strongly encourage you to write a letter to your child and send it to the agency that you worked with. If it was a private adoption through an attorney, send it to the attorney's office and ask them to put the letter in your file.

It may take years for your child to be able to financially afford to look you up. She could be waiting because she doesn't want to hurt her adoptive mother's feelings. And she may also be terrified that you'll "reject" her again.

Use your letter to tell her all about the circumstances of her adoption. Tell her about yourself, too, and any information you have about her other birth parent. Include pictures. Say everything that you've ever wanted to say to your baby. This will not only be incredibly healing for you, but will be a wonderful gift for your child.

Exercise 4

Inability to Get Pregnant

If you have been unable to get pregnant, what are your feelings about this situation? How has it affected your feelings toward your partner? Try not to make judgments or assign blame. Just record how your feelings have changed during this period of time.

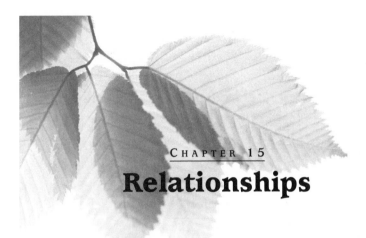

CHAPTER 15

Relationships

As we change, our relationships change, but what-
ever form they take, they can serve as mirrors of
unacknowledged parts of ourselves.

— Frances Vaughan

Someone once told me that relationships are tools for us to learn about ourselves. I didn't want to hear that! Relationships are *supposed* to be about love and romance. You grow up. You meet Mr. or Ms. Right. You fall in love, get married, and the two of you live happily ever after. Falling in love can be the most powerful experience there is. It seems to hold so many promises of the good in life. Somehow, when we're in love we believe that we'll never experience the feelings of loneliness, abandonment, fear, despair, and hopelessness again.

My own relationships all started out with a bang—that exhilarating feeling of being in love—only to quickly become painfully difficult. For so many years, I didn't know how to have a healthy relationship. I didn't know what I wanted other than to be happy.

Unfortunately, I didn't know what happiness was. One man to whom I was engaged beat me up only a little. At that time, this was happiness in comparison to another man I had previously dated who loved to bounce me off the walls. Once I started becoming healthy, I realized that getting hit or being beat up was not happiness, nor was it healthy, nor was it something that I deserved or wanted. Each relationship was a little bit healthier than the previous one.

Once I identified what physical abuse was, I moved on to emotional abuse. The emotionally abusive men I associated with also had similar beliefs about themselves. I seemed to attract men who also didn't know how to have healthy relationships. Together, we fumbled our way through, always with the shared hope of making it work. My own negative beliefs kept me going in a seemingly endless circle of painful relationships. Surprisingly, some of them were somewhat satisfying, enough to keep me there. It has taken years of unraveling my stored feelings and healing my beliefs for me to have the kind of satisfying and loving relationships I have today.

Truly, relationships do mirror back to us who we are. If we become close to another person, the feelings we are holding in our bodies will affect how we relate to each other. We may see reflected in the other person those things that we haven't allowed ourselves to see in ourselves. Or our own hidden feelings of being unworthy may attract us to people who will treat us as unworthy or even be abusive to us. Similarly, if we are carrying around a lot of resentment, anger, or rage, we may be attracted to people whose own low self-esteem draws them to us, triggering our own abusiveness. Either way, relationships have the power to help us heal.

By looking at what is mirrored back to us in a relationship, we are able to get in touch with the stored feelings that are causing our unhappiness and pain. Healing starts when, instead of blaming the other person for our pain, we look inside ourselves at the pain that is already there. This does not mean taking the blame for the other person's behavior. And it doesn't mean that it is okay to allow the other person to continue to be abusive to us. But only by healing the feelings that cause us to seek out certain kinds of relationships can we truly be free to choose the kinds of relationships that are good for us.

If there are issues in your current relationship, or if you are continually seeking out abusive relationships, it is probable that unresolved issues from the past are playing out in this battleground. Learning to interpret the reflections of yourself in others may help you get in touch with these issues, even those that are buried deep. See if any of the examples below ring true for you, or help you identify your own feelings surrounding relationships.

Example:
I feel that my husband doesn't pay enough attention to me.
Deep down inside, you may believe that you don't deserve much attention. Perhaps, if you were given a lot of attention, it would make you feel uncomfortable. Realistically, the amount of attention you are getting from your husband may be exactly as much as you need.

Example:
I feel as though I do all of the work in the relationship and I resent it.
Deep down, you may fear losing control. Your complaint may be a cover-up for your real need to control everything. Realistically, you need a man who is willing to let you do all of the work in the relationship.

Example:

My boyfriend criticizes my body, my weight, and my appearance. I am never good enough.

Your belief may be that, indeed, you are not good enough. You may have negative feelings surrounding your body, weight, and appearance. Realistically, you need a man who reflects your discontent with yourself. You could never handle a man who accepts you for who and what you are.

Example:

Throughout most of my relationships, I have felt cheated because I didn't feel that I was getting all of the love and nurturing I wanted and needed.

Your belief may have been that you didn't deserve any more than you were getting. The small amounts of love and nurturing you received didn't embarrass you or make you feel obligated. If you had received more, you might have felt suffocated.

If you are in a relationship that is causing you pain, give the mirror concept a try. Relationships are a special opportunity—a chance to see your wounds more clearly, as they are reflected back at you through your partner. The beauty of this is that it works both ways; as you begin to heal, so will your relationship. If it has outlived its purpose, it may end; but when you are ready to form a new one, it will be more nurturing and loving and less of a battleground.

You should also look at your beliefs about love and what you deserve. You might find that some beliefs that you are holding inside are that you don't deserve to have happiness, or that love is too painful, or that you don't feel worthy of the love you need. Examine those beliefs! As unromantic as this statement may be, relationships are one of our best sources for healing. Of course, they can also be wonderful, loving, nurturing, and full of joy, and ultimately that's what we want from them. The main thing to remember is that if you want to change the nature and the quality of your relationships and your life, begin by changing your beliefs about yourself.

Journal Work

Exercise 1

Naming Names

Before you begin, turn to a clean page in your journal and draw a vertical line an inch or two from the left margin. You will end up with two separate columns, narrow on the left, wide on the right. Label the left column "Names," the right one "My Unfinished Emotional Pain."

Sit comfortably. Take a few deep breaths and exhale slowly and gently. Close your eyes and ask your body, "Who's in there with whom I have unfinished business? And what is the unfinished business?"

A name may come. A face. An experience you may have forgotten. Don't just keep those names or images in your head. Write down the names and unfinished business here.

Exercise 2

Locating and Releasing the Pain

Still in a relaxed state, write down any of the physical pain that you are feeling as a result of working on Exercise 1. Do certain parts or areas of your body hurt? Acknowledge that pain to yourself by describing it in your journal. Don't discount the physical pain that may come up as the result of looking at your love relationships. You will probably discover that the pained areas are where you are storing these feelings.

Exercise 3

What You Can Do

What can you do with the pain you have? How can you release the pain from your body? Here are a few suggestions:

1. Tape a picture of the person who hurt you to the back of a chair. Pretend that this person is sitting in the chair, and tell him everything you have ever wanted to say.

2. Write a letter to the person. (You don't have to mail it.)

3. Go to a healer for your heart and whatever other body part hurts.

Exercise 4

Sexually Transmitted Diseases

Most people who have had to deal with a sexually transmitted disease have very strong feelings about it that are often hidden from conscious awareness. If you have had such a disease, write down in your journal the feelings you have around what you went through or are still going through. Describe your feelings toward the person(s) who infected you, whether you know who it was or not. Write about how other people in your life reacted when they heard that you had contracted this disease. Were they fearful? Supportive? Sympathetic? Understanding? Or did they avoid or reject you? Did they criticize or abandon you? Describe how you felt, or are still feeling, about other people's reactions.

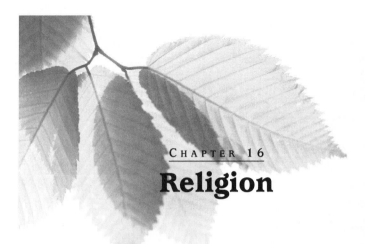

CHAPTER 16

Religion

*R*eligion in its humility restores man to his only
dignity, the courage to live by grace.

—George Santayana

There was a little girl who always looked on the bright
side of everything. No matter what was happening, she
always looked for the good. Her brothers were really tired
of her positiveness so they decided to play a trick on her.
They filled the barn with manure and sent her down there
to get something, hoping that she would get all dirty,
stinky, and sad. The little girl was gone for quite some time,
and her brothers started to worry. They thought that they
had better go and see if she was okay. They walked into the
barn and there she was, smiling and shoveling away! They
asked her what she was doing, and she replied, "With all of
this manure, there must be a pony in here somewhere!"

This story illustrates that what you find in life is all about
what you *expect* to find. This is the law of attraction. If you know,

deep inside, that you are good and wonderful and loved, then you will attract good and loving kindness into your life. If you know that goodness is within you, then you will look for it in others. The flip side of that is when you believe that you are bad or undeserving, you will tend to attract negative experiences. This, too, is the law of attraction, with a less positive outcome.

Unfortunately, many religions, or perhaps I should say religious leaders, reinforce negative feelings and beliefs that we have about ourselves. I'm not saying all religions or religious leaders do this, but many of them do.

Being a psychic and a spiritual healer for forty-two years has shown me a lot about the negativity of religions. I know about this negativity in two ways: first, through the clients I have worked with over the years; second, through the religious people who have never met me, yet believe that I am evil and what I do is evil. It's tough to turn the other cheek sometimes and allow others to have their opinions without getting into a debate.

Many religious people I have encountered love to talk about Satan. They go on and on about his powers. In a ten-minute conversation, they will mention Satan fifteen to twenty times and God once, if He's lucky! To me, it's all such a contradiction! They say they've got Jesus in their heart, yet they love to dwell on Satan. My parents taught me to pray for these people, to ask God to bless them. I have to admit, there have been many times when I have prayed for them and my heart wasn't in it!

I don't understand what gives people the right to judge others as evil or as sinners. Jesus did say "Judge them by their fruits," which I believe means that if you are going to judge people, judge them by their lives, by what they do with their gifts, their attitudes toward others, their whole essence. Get to know someone, then make your judgments based on what you have learned about her rather than on what you have heard or what you fear.

When a religion is condemnatory, harsh, shameful, and punishing, we—and our bodies—bear the results of that treatment. When we are continually reminded that we are sinners, that we are fallen, our bodies suffer. Religion is supposed to make you feel good. When it doesn't—when we inherit negative beliefs about ourselves from our religious practice or from the doctrine that is passed down from our parents—we suffer.

Until I began working on and healing my beliefs about myself, I could not have gone week after week to a church that preached what a wonderful child of God I was. For so long, I felt there was something really wrong with me and I was always afraid that people would be able to see all that bad stuff. It made me too uncomfortable to hear a lot of positive things about myself or to be told that, as a child of God, I had all the capabilities to do or be anything that I wanted. Yet, I have to admit, as Reverend Jim—former minister at the Unity Church—said in a sermon, we know deep down at the core of our being that *we are good*. And that's probably why I kept digging for that pony in my life! I had to shovel away the manure and find the goodness.

Discovering Your Goodness

Religion has the potential to be a place where it is safe to get rid of the bad feelings you are still holding on to and discover your goodness. That's what religion should be doing for all of us. It should be encouraging us to shovel away our negative beliefs and feelings about ourselves, which we have acquired along the way. It should be helping us to discover our goodness. Our holiness. Our divinity. If we are created in God's image, wouldn't that mean we have unlimited potential? That we are made out of the good in God? If you are the son or daughter of the highest Source in the Universe, you can't get much better!

Some readers are going to jump on that last statement right away! What about all of the evil people? The people who kill and abuse others? They, too, are children of God, but it's probably been lifetimes since anyone told them so. Their goodness is in there. It's just that, with all of the manure inside (negative beliefs about themselves), they probably don't even dare to look for fear they'll never find it! Their belief that they are bad is constantly reinforced by society, or by a religious system that reinforces these negative beliefs.

Look honestly at the religious system you follow. Does it reinforce your goodness or those negative beliefs that you have about yourself? Are you constantly reminded about your shortcomings? Are you told every week that you are a sinner? That you're bad? That you do not deserve happiness? What beliefs does your current religion reinforce? Can you be honest with yourself about this?

In your heart, you know if you're good or not. You know the truth about God. I remember hearing in a sermon that God told Moses, "My truth is written on your heart."

If you have discovered that your religion does reinforce your negative beliefs about yourself, it's important to start thinking about finding one that will reinforce your goodness. The problem here is that you need to start believing in it yourself. So what comes first—the chicken or the egg? It doesn't matter. What does matter is that this process of knowing your goodness begin now. Enough time has been wasted wallowing in negativity! Ask God to help direct you to a religion that will encourage you to know your goodness. I really believe in my heart that that's what God wants for you. He wants you to do everything you can to heal your pain.

Journal Work

Exercise 1

Your Present Religion

Even if you are an atheist, or haven't been to church or synagogue in years, religious teachings from your childhood can still be affecting you.

Ask yourself if your present religion reinforces your essential goodness or negative beliefs you have about yourself. The reinforcement of the positive is important to your healing. If you are holding negative feelings about yourself inside your body, this cannot be a positive influence on your health.

Write down in your journal the kinds of beliefs your place of worship reinforces and your feelings about these.

Exercise 2

Your Religious Attitudes

What do you think of when you hear the word "religion"? Even if you don't attend church or synagogue on a regular basis or think that religion has no meaning in your life, you may still be harboring bad feelings around an association with religion stemming from your childhood. If you have recently turned away from religion, you may still carry negative feelings in your body.

Record your insights, your beliefs, your memories, and your feelings about religion in your journal.

Exercise 3

Inherited Belief Systems

Sometimes the negative beliefs we find in our religious expe-riences reinforce or carry on negative beliefs or feelings that our parents taught us. Take the time to look at this possibility. If your parents were raised to believe in badness, the chances are they will raise you the same way. This cycle goes on and on until that tiny voice inside says, "Hey, I'm in here and I'm good because I was created by God!"

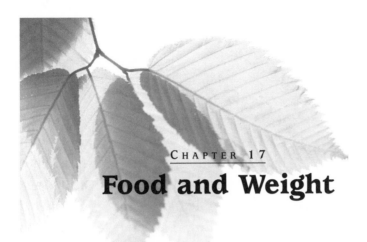

CHAPTER 17

Food and Weight

If you want to know the secret of good health, set up home in your own body, and start loving yourself when there.

—John W. Travis, MD

Some years ago I met a woman who was the sales manager for a well-known weight loss program. She told me that she had just won a cruise for having the highest sales record in her region. Since I had struggled with weight issues for most of my life, it was very difficult for me to sit and listen to her celebrate her achievement. She talked about weight loss as a product, much as one would discuss cars or computers. Not once did she mention the emotional aspects of being overweight; to her, it was business, plain and simple. All of those overweight people were just figures in the books at the end of each month.

But I know differently. After years and years of working as a psychic and healer and hearing the conflicts, confusion, and suffering people have surrounding their weight, dieting on my own, joining weight loss programs, working out at health clubs, buying workout tapes, taking diet pills, surviving on protein drinks, and reading all of the latest diet books, I know that most weight loss issues are due not to overeating but to unresolved emotions.

It has always been difficult for me to express my feelings; it is much easier to stuff them down with food. This way only I suffer, and the person I am angry with or afraid of does not. When I was little, food comforted me. I often felt lonely as a child and have fond memories of Twinkies filling that void. Oreo cookies helped when I felt afraid or sad. Many times, when I was little and hurt myself, someone gave me a cookie and it always made me feel better! Now, wanting to feel better is strongly associated with eating food.

I recently heard an advertisement on the radio for an eating disorders clinic in Minneapolis. It was a word association test in which the narrator, usually a therapist, said a word and the person taking the test said the first thing that came to mind. The commercial went something like this:

Narrator Word Association	Client Response
afraid	cookies
sad	ice cream
alone	pizza
mad	hot dogs
panic	potato chips
overwhelmed	doughnuts
anxious	Snickers candy bar
rage	licorice

Food isn't just food; food serves an emotional purpose! Food is a source of comfort, and it's what we turn to when we feel empty, lonely, afraid, sad, angry, overwhelmed, or anxious. Food silences those negative feelings and beliefs, if only for a little while, and yes, food makes us feel better.

Of course, that is why despite the billion-dollar weight loss industry in this country, we are not conquering our weight problem. How many times have you read about the ridiculously high percentage of people who lose weight, only to gain it back within the first year? We watch shows like *The Biggest Loser,* and root for those poor souls—even as we fear for them. How likely are they to keep the weight off, once the cameras stop rolling? Once they no longer have the support of a peer group, and a home audience rooting them on, will they be able to conquer the battle of the bulge?

The Emotions behind Eating

I have come to believe that being thin will not come from going on diets for the rest of my life. The most successful weight loss program I was ever on was one that incorporated an emotional support group. We met weekly (until the program was suspended) and helped each other identify and cope with emotional issues around our weight gain and loss.

I began to realize that whatever food did for me as a child, it was doing for me as an adult. This realization led me to ask myself: What is my behavior around food? When do I turn to it? No matter what time of day it is, if I feel empty, lonely, afraid, sad, angry, overwhelmed, or anxious, food is my comforter. It isn't expensive or time-consuming to get. When I need a quick fix, all I need to do is jump in the car and drive to the nearest convenience store. Now I have learned that in order to keep the weight off, I have to find ways to express my feelings. I have to work on feeling safe. Unsafe feelings or vulnerability are major triggers for wanting to eat.

While people need to cut back on caloric intake to get those pounds off, they also must look at what the food does for them emotionally. Understanding these issues—identifying the reason behind binge eating or yo-yo dieting—can help you develop better eating habits and finally keep the weight off for good.

If you've struggled with weight loss issues for a long time, it may be because you are getting emotional payoffs from being overweight. For example, suppose you are shy or have a deep-down fear of intimacy. Fat may be a buffer between you and the world—a way of protecting yourself from other people. If you are big, people won't get too close. If you are an introvert, a person who needs and likes lots of time alone throughout the day, the extra weight is your way of making sure that you have enough space to breathe. Being overweight also offers this excuse: "I don't have any clothes that fit, so I will have to stay home."

If you are insecure, extra weight may make you feel more powerful. If you are trying to learn how to share your feelings with others or how to be more spontaneous and less controlled, or just want others to pay you some attention, it is helpful to feel *big.* You might feel that if you are physically thin, people won't take you seriously because you look fragile. Diagnose and treat the underlying issue, and you solve the food problem.

A young woman named Rachel came to see me for a weight problem. Since childhood, her eating had been out of control. She had joined a twelve-step group for eating disorders, but said her weight seemed to be getting worse rather than better.

While channeling a healing for her, I looked inside psychically and saw a little girl running from a woman (her mother) who was attempting to strangle her. I saw her father nearby, ignoring her cries for help. I could see, too, that he had been extremely cruel to her, both verbally and physically.

John told me that the only way Rachel felt safe was to get as big as possible so no one would ever hurt her again. Since the birth of her baby brother, she had felt invisible to her family and wanted to be bigger so they would notice her, too. Now an adult, in addition to her weight problem, she had serious issues around intimacy and trust, especially pertaining to men. Her only way of coping with these unresolved issues and feelings was to overeat. The more she overate, the worse she felt about herself.

If you are overweight, chances are you are very angry with yourself and your body. Remember, the abusive way you talk to yourself will not change your relationship to food or help you lose weight. You are going to have to go within and search out the real issues—what is really eating away at you inside. Use your weight problem to get to the heart of your negative feelings and beliefs.

Changing Behavioral Patterns

Generally, the people who are most successful are those who combine a supportive weight loss program with a thorough exploration of the emotional purpose of food in their lives.

As you look inside, you may become aware of behavioral patterns that are affecting your attitude about food and weight loss. Whatever behavior patterns you perceive, remember that you can change them.

If you find that you overeat or keep weight on to protect yourself, you can start now to find ways of providing safety for yourself. You can remove yourself from threatening situations. It is important to stay present, focused on the *now*, and to pray for the strength you need to get out of any frightening or painful situations. If you feel threatened, call friends and get their support. If you are in a situation where harm can come to you, call 911. Don't hesitate. There are community support groups and other resources to help you with virtually any threatening situation. As adults, we can protect ourselves. We no longer have to be victims!

Many experts on weight management say that it is virtually impossible to heal the issues we have around weight without help from at least one other supportive person. That person might be a close friend who is struggling with issues very similar to yours and is also willing to look inside for solutions. Or it might be a therapist, healer, or support group that will provide you with the outside help that will work for you.

Love Yourself

Yes, I know. It is difficult to love yourself when you don't like your physical appearance. But if when you look in the mirror you see a person who is heavier than you want to be, remember that there are reasons for your weight problem. It has literally nothing to do with your lack of will power, so don't wallow in guilt the next time someone tells you that all you need is a little self-control. Remind yourself that it's your body and you don't need other people's judgments.

Journal Work

I believe it is your wounded inner child that is responsible for most of your weight problems.

Your inner child rebels against being placed on restricted diets. It hates being told no, especially if it heard this throughout its childhood. Now that it is an adult and can have whatever it wants, it does.

It wants treats when its feelings have been hurt. It wants and needs nurturing, and if food was how it was nurtured, it doesn't want to give it up.

If you are a workaholic, the only form of "fun" your inner child might have is visits to the Dairy Queen, a whole bag of M&M's, or Ben and Jerry's at midnight.

Exercise 1

See How You Eat

Take a good look at the way you eat. Do you eat like an adult giving your body good nutrition, or do you eat like a child? I have a friend who still eats the way he did when he was a child. Sixty-two years old and he lives on Jello, hot dogs, Kool-aid, and cookies!

Exercise 2

Food and Your Inner Child

If you are struggling with a weight problem, I want you to spend some quality time with your inner child. Get out its crayons and coloring tablet and ask it to tell you what kinds of food it particularly likes and what makes that food special. Ask it how it feels when you go on a diet. Ask it if it eats when it's mad or sad.

Also, ask it if it uses your extra weight as protection against mean people.

And finally, ask it how it would feel if you were thin.

Please be patient with your inner child as it dialogues with you, and don't become critical. If your inner child is feeling vulnerable all the time, and weight and certain foods are the only thing that make it feel safe, then you are not going to lose the weight until these issues get resolved—no matter how long that takes.

The next time you go to grab for food that isn't necessarily healthy for you or your waistline, grab your writing tablet first, and ask your inner child what it *really* needs.

Hopefully, you will get the insight you're looking for to end the cycle of weight loss/weight gain.

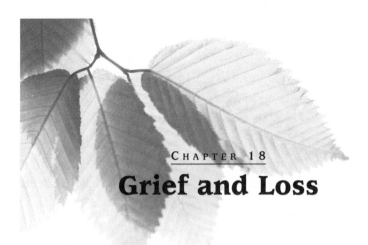

Chapter 18

Grief and Loss

A llow yourself your grieving. Allow it to express in whatever way feels right to you. Grieving is the way we heal the loss we feel for someone we love.
—Deborah Duda

Every year between Thanksgiving and Christmas until the age of thirty-five, I would feel a deep sense of loss inside. A deep, deep sadness. It was as though I had lost something really important. No matter how excited I was about the holidays, no matter how busy I was preparing for the holiday season, I would invariably feel a deep gnawing for the entire month. It was as if I had once had something very special and had lost it. Some years I would go into such a deep depression that I would tell my family I just couldn't participate in the holidays. Feeling the heavy sense of loss of something that I didn't even understand, plus baking, shopping, wrapping presents, and tree-trimming were all just way too much for me.

There was also another feeling that was hard to cope with, a feeling as if I was once special but that something had happened and that specialness had been taken away. Every year I would mentally prepare myself. I would say affirmations, thinking that if I was in a good place mentally before December, maybe that would ward off my sadness. Some years I went into therapy, hoping that talking about it in advance would ward it off. No matter what I did, that deep sense of loss would begin all over again.

My wedding date was December 16, 1983. I was sure that when the time approached that year I would be so excited I just wouldn't fall into that all-too-familiar heaviness. But, sure enough, the first week in December rolled around and out came the tears! I always felt so little, as if I was a three-year-old again. I felt vulnerable, afraid, alone, and confused.

What the heck was this all about? Here I was, thirty-five years old, and this damn bogeyman would not go away. I prayed for help once again and soon afterward, I felt intuitively that I should call my mother. At first, my intellect got in the way and said not to bother her with this again, that she'd heard me talk about it for years. We had talked about it so much that there wasn't much more to say. Despite this, I did feel the inner nudging again, so I gave her a call.

Something was different this time. Maybe it was because I finally knew how to express my feelings more clearly or that it was just time for it to be revealed . . . I'm not sure. Maybe it was because this time I said more to my mom than just how sad and empty and depressed I felt, which is what I had always said in the past. Being in therapy was helping me to identify my feelings and talk about them more clearly.

I told my mom that I was feeling that heavy sense of loss again and didn't want it overshadowing the wedding. I just needed to talk through each feeling with her. I needed to tell her it felt as if I was once really special but that this feeling had just vanished from my life. I told her that I felt as if I wanted to go find what I had lost. It felt as if one day, long ago, I had been okay and the next day I was all alone.

As I was sharing these feelings with her, I was sobbing like a baby, which is what I did every December. Feeling the heaviness of my sense of loss and crying, my mom listened carefully to me and suddenly realized what was going on.

She told me that from the time I was a baby until I was four, a person who had dearly loved me was my grandpa. She said he would come over every day to see me. He always read to me, taught me things, and treated me as very special. When I turned three, he discovered he had cancer and wasn't able to come over every day for our visits. Also, I had a new baby brother. My life was changing.

Mom told me that right after Thanksgiving that year he got very sick, and in December he died. I never saw him after that Thanksgiving. She said they didn't know how to explain death to a four-year-old, so they just never said anything about Grandpa. As a little four-year-old, all I knew was that my best friend, who had been by my side every day of my life and who had treated me as very special, never came back. I may have felt that I did something wrong or that his going away had something to do with the new baby. I don't know how I felt or reasoned it out in my childhood mind. We had never talked about my grandfather's death, but all my feelings about that loss were still in there! Every December they reminded me of my loss.

That night and for the next few days, I let myself feel all of it. Whenever my intellect tried to take over and tell me that enough is enough, I told it to stop trying to interfere. I wanted to be free from the sadness. I talked to my grandfather, pretended he was there, and thanked him for all he had given me while he was here.

It felt as if a tremendous healing took place over that three-day period. It was wonderful. It has been twenty-five years since that time, and I can honestly say that I have not experienced another black December in all that time.

I can't emphasize enough the importance of getting those feelings of loss out of your body. In my case, those feelings always manifested in my body as digestion problems and headaches throughout the month of December. It was as physically difficult as it was emotionally trying for me during that time of year, until I discovered the truth about the close, loving relationship I had with my grandfather.

Throughout our lives, we suffer from many different kinds of losses: the death of a loved one; the breakup of a relationship; the pain of a divorce; or the loss of a home through natural disaster, a fire, or moving to another city. We experience the loss of a job, our health, money, success, a pet, material possessions, teachers, or our youth.

Everyone experiences loss. It's a part of life. When we suffer from a physical injury, we are given time to heal. People send us cards and flowers. Sometimes we are even paid to take time off so we can heal. Unfortunately, when we suffer an emotional injury, such as the loss of a loved one, not only are we expected to rise above it and get back to work, sometimes people don't know what to say to us, so they don't say anything. On top of feeling the loss, we feel terribly alone.

For most of us, loss and grief generate a multitude of feelings. Some of these stem from our inability to know what to do. We don't know how much time we're allowed to grieve. We feel guilty if we don't grieve "appropriately," yet what is appropriate? Is it okay to feel pain, cry, yell, scream, be numb, get angry, play sad songs, wallow in memories, get mad at God?

For many of us, the response is to do whatever we can to make the pain go away as fast as possible. We search for ways to distract us from our pain. Or we pretend we're over our pain so that (a) we don't have to feel our feelings; and (b) others don't have to be *bothered* with our feelings.

Loss and Healing

The bottom line is that there is nothing worse than the pain of loss. The bad news is that it hurts like hell and there is no magic pill to relieve it. Even if your doctor gives you a "magic" pill, the pain is still inside and needs to be released. The good news is that by going inside we may also release other issues, other negative emotions that have been bottled up. As difficult as it may seem at the time, loss really does promote healing.

Time and *going into* the pain is what brings about the cure. When you have a pain, whether it's physical or emotional, take a deep breath and lean into the pain. Don't resist it. The less you resist the pain, the quicker you will come out of it.

Feel the loss. Feel the emptiness. Feel the aloneness. You will not die if you allow yourself to feel it. It will be less stressful to your body if you feel it rather than resist it. Once you allow yourself to go into the pain, your healing process begins. Closing the door on a chapter in our lives is difficult but not impossible. We do survive loss.

Loss and Physical Pain

Perhaps you're grieving a loss right now. If so, do you have any physical pain? Where in your body is it being stored? You may not be able to answer this question right away, and that's okay. It is enough to start this process of letting go by giving some thought to the losses you have had in your life and whether or not you allowed yourself to adequately grieve those losses.

The reason I ask about physical pain is that there's a good chance that your body is acting it out in some way, if you're not emotionally grieving the loss. For example, some time ago, my minister died. He had been a mentor of mine for quite a while. When he was diagnosed with cancer, it was really hard for me to accept. His death shortly thereafter was even harder. I didn't want to feel the loss emotionally.

I was afraid that if I went into the pain of his death, I would be devastated and wouldn't be able to come out of it. On the day of his memorial service, I had the most excruciating lower back pain. I ended up in the emergency room of the hospital. The doctor said there was something wrong with my kidneys, but had no idea what it could be. Kidneys have to do with elimination. I believe that my kidneys were saying, Eliminate this pain. Let it out. Stop holding it in. I spent the rest of the day crying about his death. By the end of the day, the lower back pain was gone. These unresolved feelings really do cause us physical pain!

If you discover in doing the journal work at the end of this chapter that you have not grieved over some of your losses, I strongly suggest that you take some time and write down all of your feelings about each loss in your journal. If you feel fearful of becoming overwhelmed with emotion, I recommend that you call a local hospital and see if grief groups are available. If not, ask them whom they would recommend, or ask your doctor or therapist. Grieving does not need to go on forever. When you really face the loss and feel it, when you fully express your feelings about it, you become free to move back into life. By pretending that the feelings of grief are not inside, you become imprisoned by your own feelings. You are not free to live your life spontaneously with an open heart. Pray for the courage to complete your grief and free yourself from the pain of loss. It's worth it!

Journal Work

Exercise 1

Identifying the Loss

In your journal, make two columns of approximately the same size by drawing a vertical line down the middle of the page. Label the left column "My Losses," the right column "How I Did or Didn't Respond."

Now, in the corresponding column, write down the losses you have had in your lifetime. Go into as much or as little detail as you wish. Then, in the right column, describe how you responded to that loss. If you felt numb about the loss, or simply didn't respond, write that.

Exercise 2

Losses Experienced from Deep Within

Divide a blank page in your journal with a vertical line down the middle, labeling the left column "My Child's Losses" and the right column "How I (When a Child) Responded to the Loss."

Using your nondominant hand, ask your inner child to write about the losses it has suffered. Remember, this is a child's response. Your inner child's answers will be different from your own. The goal here is to get all those losses out of your body and onto paper.

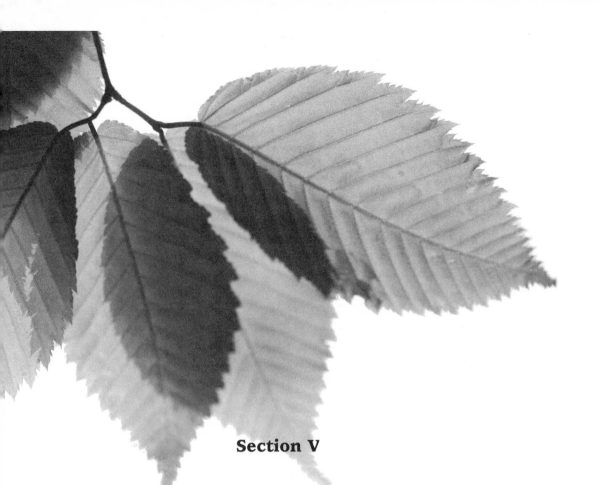

Section V

Getting Better

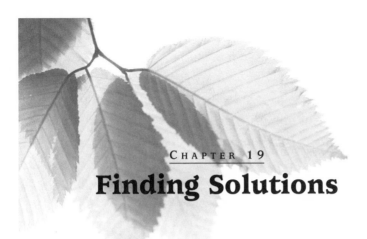

CHAPTER 19

Finding Solutions

The wisdom of nature can give us all the answers to our day-to-day problems and show us the way to heal ourselves.

—Gerald G. Jampolsky, MD, and Diane Cirincione

If you are anything like me, you are anxious to discover the quickest solutions to any problem or question. But the first thing I have to tell you is not to be in too much of a hurry. At the same time, don't lose your passion to get better. You are already on your way. You've realized that something isn't right inside, and you are reading books about healing.

Your mind and body are in the process of shifting from the old way of thinking, feeling, and being into a new way—and the key word here is "process." I've always hated that word. It means there are going to be different stages and that relief from the pain is going to take time. But that is what we must accept on the healing journey.

Asking your Higher Power for help is very important. Simply

ask each day that you continue to have the strength, courage, and desire to grow out of the old pain and into freedom.

Many of us get stuck because we lack courage. We fear change and the unknown. Who will we be, after we get rid of the old stories, the old way of thinking and reacting? Will people still like us if we turn in our victim roles to find freedom for ourselves? You may have already encountered people who will do everything they can to keep you the way you are even though you want to change. Your getting well may very well threaten those closest to you. But you don't need to get caught in this trap.

Write the following words on a piece of paper:

This is my journey, my turn for freedom. My time for healing.

Keep these words close to you—pinned on your bulletin board at work, folded in your wallet, or tacked to your refrigerator. Recite these words as your mantra, or incorporate them into your daily meditation practice, if you have one. Let them remind you that it is time to focus on your freedom, peace of mind, and health.

Following are ten solutions to help you heal—but remember, healing can only begin if you give yourself permission to focus on yourself. If you can do that—if you can remember how important you are—healing your emotions will have a tremendous effect on your body, your mind, your soul, your relationships, your work, your spirituality, your life!

Solution 1: Finding a Good Doctor

The first step, if you are in physical pain, is to find a good doctor. Do you have one who listens to you and who will spend quality time with you? One who returns your calls? One who treats you with respect? If you don't have a wonderful doctor, it is time to shop around. Don't get caught up in false loyalty. You don't have to go to a doctor just because your parents did or because she is your neighbor. Remember, this is your body. It runs like a magnificent machine when all systems are go. When all systems aren't go, you need help! Take your body to someone you really trust. You need someone who will listen to what you have to say.

Being sick is hard enough without an insensitive doctor telling you that your symptoms are in your head. Please don't think you need to put up with a doctor who makes you feel bad about yourself. There are many qualified physicians out there who went into medicine because they want to help people. Remember, if your body hurts, something is wrong! Don't just wait for days or weeks for the pain to go away. If it persists, your body is talking to you. It wants you to listen!

Here are some suggestions concerning doctors and your health.

1. **You must fight for yourself!** If you are in physical pain, call your doctor or go in to see her. If your doctor doesn't return your call, call back. Don't let a nurse put you off. When you do get in to see your doctor, tell her all the symptoms that you are having. She is not going to know what you "kind of mean." Your doctor needs to hear the whole story. All of your symptoms. Your doctor's job is to help you fix your body, so you've got to describe what's hurting you.

2. **Try not to treat the doctor as if he is God.** Doctors are not God, and giving them that kind of power is just going to get in the way of your getting the help you need. If you happen to find a doctor who wants to be treated like God, go find another one. You're not there to boost his ego. You're there for your body's sake.

3. **Don't think of yourself as a "bother."** I have heard so many clients say that they don't want to bother their doctor with the pains that they're having or the fears they're experiencing. If the heat went out in your house, would you hesitate to call your local gas company because you don't want to hassle them? If your doctor has a busy schedule, that is not your responsibility. If she is hassled, it is up to her and her office staff to make some changes. It is your doctor's professional responsibility to provide you with the service you require; if she is not doing that, it's time for you to find someone who will.

4. **Remember, this is your one and only body.** No one else knows what is going on in your body other than you and your doctor, so keep that line of communication open and make sure you get your needs met.

Solution 2: Professional Support

You have been asked throughout this book to look at and write down all of your feelings, beliefs, memories, and pain. This has helped you to release the emotional blocks and confront many of them for the first time. A therapist can help you work through the final stages of healing.

Ask friends, relatives, or your doctor to recommend someone who is not judgmental or shaming. You need someone who believes that your health problems are connected to emotional issues. You need someone who believes that your past does affect your future and who will encourage you to go back as often as necessary to get it all out.

Look for a therapist who is relatively busy, and who will not hang on to you simply because he needs the business. You also need someone who will help you as quickly as possible. Ask God or the Universe to direct you to just the right person. You also need to do your part in looking. But you will be amazed at how easily you will be led to the right person if you just ask.

Above all, don't let money or pride keep you stuck. Your body's health and healing process should be at the top of your list of priorities! Don't get stuck in worrying about whether or not your insurance will cover the costs. It isn't as if you can turn this body in and get another one. Get what your body needs in the way of help, and if you end up with a bill, slowly pay it off. Bills are a fact of life. They motivate us to go to work, so don't let bills be your excuse for not getting well. This is your healing process. Many therapists have a sliding fee scale, which means that they charge according to your income. Many government offices provide free counseling. Don't sabotage your healing process because of money issues! Ask for help.

Once you enter therapy, take all that you have written from the exercises in this book and share it with your therapist. Sort through it all, feel it, talk it out, and, hopefully, leave all of your pain there. That's the therapist's job. A therapist's office is like the emotional sanitation department. Dump it all at the emotional garbage station!

When I left my therapist's office each week, I would ask her for an assignment, something that I could work on in between visits. Even though I didn't always want to do what she suggested, I forced myself, and it always helped. For example, her suggestion that I share one of my feelings each day with at least one person was a difficult task for me, but she said it would help me feel more connected to people and life, and she was right.

Ask your therapist for ideas about what you can do in between visits, so that you feel more in charge of your healing process and be sure that it is progressing. Make a series of appointments, so you can stay in the flow. Remember, even though you now have help, you are still responsible for your own healing.

Lifeworks Clinics

Lifeworks is a program designed to help people discover and work through their self-defeating patterns of living, and I can't say enough good things about it. It provides help and a safe environment where you can take a good, hard look at your family of origin—your roots. It is especially helpful for those who are: (1) struggling with issues of compulsive, addictive, or self-defeating coping patterns; (2) struggling with codependency and related intimacy issues; (3) adult children of alcoholics or from other types of dysfunctional family backgrounds; and (4) survivors of emotional, physical, and sexual abuse or neglect.

Lifeworks creates a unique and safe environment where you can allow yourself to feel your feelings, let the inner volcanoes explode if they need to, and feel good about it. My experiences at a Lifeworks clinic saved my life, helping me break free of old, destructive patterns to live a freer, more healthful life.

If you are feeling stuck and are tired of it, I strongly suggest that you go to www.clearlife.com and find out their schedule for upcoming clinics. If you are not able to travel to them, ask if they know of a similar program in your area.

Solution 3: Twelve-Step Groups

I've talked about the importance of finding a personal therapist to help you with emotional issues. I've talked about finding a competent doctor to help with the physical symptoms. What we need to look at next are the spiritual needs of your body and soul. It's important that you not try to do all of this work by yourself. Consider getting involved in a support group. The twelve-step programs are a great beginning.

What Are the Twelve Steps?

The Twelve Steps of AA are relatively simple, straightforward guidelines that can help us work through almost any kind of habit or behavior that has us stuck:

1. We admitted we were powerless over alcohol—that our lives had become unmanageable.

2. We came to believe that a Power greater than our selves could restore us to sanity.

3. We made a decision to turn our will and our lives over to the care of God as we understood Him.

4. We made a searching and fearless moral inventory of ourselves.

5. We admitted to God, to ourselves, and to another human being the exact nature of our wrongs.

6. We were entirely ready to have God remove all these defects of character.

7. We humbly asked Him to remove our shortcomings.

8. We made a list of all persons we had harmed, and became willing to make amends to them all.

9. We made direct amends to such people wherever possible, except when to do so would injure them or others.

10. We continued to take personal inventory and when we were wrong promptly admitted it.

11. We sought through prayer and meditation to improve our conscious contact with God as we understood Him, praying only for knowledge of His will for us and the power to carry that out.

12. Having had a spiritual awakening as the result of these Steps, we tried to carry this message to alcoholics, and to practice these principles in all our affairs.

Twelve-step groups, based on these guidelines, are spiritual in nature. You do not need to be an alcoholic to live these steps, as they have been adopted by all kinds of groups with different needs. Check online or in your local white pages for the twelve-step group that sounds as if it would fit your needs best. If you can't find anything listed in your area, I would suggest you look up the number for your local Alcoholics Anonymous Central Intergroup Office. They usually have the numbers of other twelve-step groups in their area. Here's the latest list:

Alcoholics Anonymous

Al-Anon (for spouses or loved ones of alcoholics or drug addicts)

Cocaine Anonymous

Codependents Anonymous

Co-Survivors of Incest Anonymous

Emotions Anonymous

Families Anonymous

Gamblers Anonymous

Narcotics Anonymous

Overeaters Anonymous

Parents Anonymous

Pill Anonymous

Recovering Couples Anonymous

Sex Addicts Anonymous

Sex and Love Addicts Anonymous

Sexaholics Anonymous

Co-Sa (for loved ones of sex addicts)

Shoplifters Anonymous

Smokers Anonymous

Shoppers Anonymous

Spenders Anonymous

Survivors of Incest Anonymous

Twelve Steps for Christian Living

Twelve Steps for Spiritual Growth

Women for Sobriety

You will want to check a group out first before going in and telling your whole life story. First, get a sense of how the group feels. Ask for literature. Most twelve-step groups run strictly on one-dollar donations from each member weekly. There are no dues or fees. If you can't afford a dollar, no one will hassle you or judge you. There are no memberships. There is no test to take in order to get in. As a matter of fact, all that you need is a desire to get better.

The reason for the word "anonymous" is that in true twelve-step groups your anonymity is protected. Everything you say stays at the meeting.

Groups set up by gender (only for men or only for women) can also be really helpful, and I highly recommend attending one. You will learn more about yourself by listening to other people of the same gender talk about themselves. It's scary to sit in with a group of strangers and talk about who you are. But, remember, newcomers are strangers for only a short time.

Solution 4: Asking for a Healing

This solution is different from the rest in that there is very little you need to do other than to reach out for help and then allow it to come to you.

Laying-on-of-hands healing, the type of healing I do and which I have referred to throughout this book, is very straightforward. I've been doing it for forty-two years, and it's so simple that most people have trouble believing it works. They try to complicate it with rituals, sounds, methods, or step-by-step instructions—as if God's amazing healing energy isn't enough on it's own! My first book, *Hands That Heal,* gives complete instructions for channeling healing energy.

Absentee Healing

Over the years, I've also become familiar with a form of healing called absentee healing. In this type of healing, the healer does not need to be in the same room with a person in order to heal. The healer prays for the person to be healed, and a healing takes place. One example of such a healing is the Bible story in which a father goes to Jesus and asks him to come to his home and heal his daughter. Jesus tells the man that because of his faith, his daughter has been healed and that all he needs to do is go home and be with her.

At www.Echobodine.com, I have developed an absentee healing program called Healing Pen Pals. You simply email us your name, location, and the type of healing you request. Our coordinators then assign one of our hundred healers the task of sending you healing energy every day for two weeks. If at the end of two weeks you still need more, the healer will send healing for another two weeks. There is no charge for this service. All we ask is that you let us know after the first two weeks how you're doing. In the past two years, we have served close to four thousand people, and, as the testimonials on the site reveal, the results have been amazing.

If you don't have email, you can still take advantage of this service. Send a letter with your name, age, city that you live in, and what you would like a healing for, to:

Healing Pen Pals
c/o Echo Bodine
P.O. Box 19488
Minneapolis, MN 55419
United States

Let us help you to heal that pain.

Solution 5: t.t.G.

Another solution I especially like is to t.t.G. (talk to God). I don't even want to say the p-word (prayer) because so many people get stuck there. They see the word and immediately stiffen up and think of some formalized, ritualistic prayer they learned as a child.

I don't believe God wants to hear some formalized prayer. I believe God wants to hear from you—your thoughts, feelings, needs, desires, wants, fears, tears, and anxieties. I believe that whatever you have to say, God wants to hear it!

When I first got into recovery, the idea of talking to God was a little scary for me, as it is for a lot of other newcomers to a spiritual way of life. At my church, someone came up with the idea of a God Box. Whenever any of us had a need to talk to God or had a prayer request, we would write it down and put it in the God Box. The youth group at our church has a God Can. I like that idea better than a God Box because it's a reminder that "God can."

Writing letters to God has become a great way for me to share with Him all that goes on with me. It's also a good way to get to know myself. I have saved my letters to God throughout the years, and it's fun to look back at them and see my progress. It's also been a good way to build faith and to see that the prayers do get answered.

Fortunately for me, not all prayers are answered with a yes, including things that I thought I just had to have, such as relationships with men, certain jobs, or places to live. I have learned that what I think I must have is sometimes not that good for me in the long run, and in the end, God really does know best.

Step 11 of AA's twelve-step program says: "We sought through prayer and meditation to improve our conscious contact with God as we understand Him, praying only for knowledge of His will for us and the power to carry that out."

I have learned, after some resistance, to pray for knowledge of God's will for me. This has always turned out to be better than my will for myself. Sometimes my issues about unworthiness and undeservingness get in the way. What I want or see for myself often comes up short of God's will for me.

There was a man in my life that I really wanted a relationship with. I pleaded with God to please let it happen. I was sure that man was all I needed to be happy and feel complete. This went on for two years. We would date, but as soon as we would get close, he'd go away physically and emotionally. I couldn't see how bad he was for me. I look back at all of those old, pleading prayers. Thank God I didn't get what I thought I had to have! God has always had something better in mind, so I have come to a place in my prayers where I ask for God's will to be done. This doesn't mean that I don't ask for my desires, dreams, wants, and needs, but because experience has taught me that God's will is much greater, I always end my requests with, "Thy will be done, not mine." That way, I've said what's on my mind and still sought my highest good!

People often ask me how I pray. Some seem surprised that I talk to God as I would my best friend. I need God to know me. I need to feel that connection to my Source. That oneness. All throughout the day, I talk to God about everything: decisions that need to be made, feelings that I have, fears that I bump up against. I ask for guidance all the time. No, I don't get down on my knees. I used to, but I don't think that it matters to God what position I'm in when I'm talking to Him. I think that what's most important is the communication. It helps me feel grounded, centered.

I think that it's so important to our daily peace of mind and sense of direction to talk to God. I can't imagine the chaos if I were trying to figure this out all by myself. What about you? How comfortable are you with talking to God? If you haven't talked to God for a long time or if you have never talked to Him, don't let that stop you! God didn't go away. God doesn't hold grudges or keep score. God is there for you to talk to about yourself, your life, your troubles, your dreams. Whatever concerns you, concerns God.

Some of you may only feel comfortable talking to God by starting out with a ritualistic, formalized prayer. That is fine, but please don't stop there! I know that if you haven't done this for a while, it can be scary or feel strange. Just go slowly. Be gentle with yourself. Tell God that you're afraid, nervous. Every day try to make some conversation. After a while, you will sense the presence of God. The feeling of God. You'll know God is listening. As time passes, you'll talk more and more. Developing this relationship is a process, just like everything else. Just start . . . talking to God . . . and when you're done talking, go on to the next solution, l.t.G.—Listen to God!

Solution 6: l.t.G.

After you spend time talking to God, you need to give God some time to talk back. Praying is talking to God or the Universe, and meditating is listening to God or the Universe. Meditation is a means by which our minds and bodies become calm. The purpose is to get your mind on the outer world and focus on your inner world—that inner sanctuary. While it may seem impossible at times to become calm, it really isn't! There are wonderful meditation books on the market or meditation classes you can attend. Many bookstores also carry CDs that you can listen to that will teach you how to meditate. At first, I would caution you to *keep it simple.*

You need to take yourself away from the "busyness" of the world and become still, even if it's just for five minutes. Some people have a special place set up in their homes or offices where they meditate. Some need to go to a church or a meditation center. Some like to meditate in a natural setting, such as a garden, a park, the woods, or the seashore. Remember, whatever works for you is right.

Personally, I don't have a specific place set up for meditation. In the mornings, before I climb out of bed, I lie there in that very relaxed state and ask God what I need to know or do for that day. Images come to me. So do feelings. Inspirations, too, of people to call or places to go. Direction. Throughout the day, I keep one ear open to the world and one ear open to God. My former minister, Rev. Don Clark, said in a sermon, "God doesn't shout . . . God speaks softly, so don't expect your guidance to come thundering in from on high. Keep an open ear to God at all times." God speaks to us through our intuition. You might feel an inner nudge to go to the grocery store, and that's where you will find the answer that you've been looking for. Our answers come in so many ways: through our thoughts, our friends, family members, and others. God certainly isn't limited in how He/She can get answers to us. That makes it fun!

People tend to make meditation more complicated than it needs to be. Simply put, it is taking the time to listen to the Universe, God, your Source, or whatever you want to call it, so that you feel centered and directed. You may find it easier in the beginning to focus on something other than yourself. Consider purchasing a CD or meditation book. Listen to the CD or read the book for that day. Periodically throughout the day, think back to the words of your meditation. Become calm again.

Some people get so intimidated by the idea of meditation that they never try it. They are afraid they won't do it right. Don't get caught up in that kind of thinking. Just take some time each day to focus on your Source—whatever you call your Higher Power. Talk, and then sit in the silence and listen. Don't worry if nothing comes; there's always tomorrow.

Solution 7: Alternative Healthcare

So much has changed in the healthcare field since the first edition of this book was published in 1993. Many hospitals today are incorporating alternative methods of healthcare, and I'm so happy to see this. Some are offering laying-on-of-hands healing, acupuncture, biofeedback, and other means of therapeutic modalities.

There is so much that the alternative healthcare field has to offer in the way of helping you heal, and I would strongly suggest you take a look at what is available to you in your area. Psychics, astrologers, healers, masseuses, chiropractors, osteopaths, numerologists, herbalists, nutritionists, rolfers, and shamans are just a few that come to mind.

I have one suggestion when seeking out alternative healthcare, and that is to ask your friends if they know of or have heard of a reputable person. I only go to people that I have been referred to, and I always get the full scoop from anyone who gives me a referral. What kind of service does this person provide? What can I expect from the session? How many sessions might it take before I see results? Do they take insurance? What is their fee?

Most people who are involved in the alternative healing arts in one form or another are on a spiritual path and truly want to be helpful in your healing process, but there are some who are not sincere and are only in it for the money or the prestige of "being a healer." Whenever you are seeking medical help, always run it by your intuition to see if the person feels like a good fit for you. No more victim, remember?

Solution 8: A Positive Attitude

As soon as you ask if there is another way of doing things, you are on your way to discovering other possibilities and choices. In order for us to be open to other choices or solutions, we need to be willing to let go of being victims. Thinking like, feeling like, and believing that you are a victim may be one of the most difficult beliefs you will have to work through. It is so much easier to point the finger at other people in your life and say, "It's your fault that I am the way I am," or "It's your fault I'm having a bad day," or, "If only my spouse would get his act together, then I would be happy."

It's been difficult for me to admit that I play and wear the victim role very easily. It seems so automatic to start blaming as soon as something goes wrong. Why is it so much easier to point a finger of blame than to take responsibility for what happens in our lives? I think that a big part of it comes from so many of us being afraid of making mistakes. To have to admit that we made a mistake can sometimes be more than we feel we can do.

I have a friend who chooses to believe the negative side of everything. He says that then he won't be discouraged when life lets him down. I know there are plenty of people who live by that same philosophy. Unfortunately, when life is good to them, they seem disappointed too. That's how it is with my friend. Whenever something wonderful happens in his life, he can barely talk about it. When he finally does share the good news, he ends the story with, "We'll see." This usually means, "We'll see if it is really going to be good. We'll see if this really isn't just a hassle wrapped in a pretty package. We'll see if life isn't just messing with me."

One thing that I have learned about life is that it invariably gives me what I'm expecting. It's true. I may be praying for a new car but if I am expecting to get a used car with lots of mileage, that's what the Universe will deliver. It seems to go back to those beliefs again! What we believe to be true is how it's going to happen.

The Power of Belief

Most of us have heard the saying, "I'll believe it when I see it." But a few years ago, while talking to my minister, I made a slip of the tongue and said, "I'll see it when I believe it." We both had a good laugh with that one! But there was also an important truth expressed in my mistake. Our beliefs really do tend to determine what we see! If I believe that work is going to be crummy, it will be crummy. If I believe I'm going to gain weight, I will. If I believe I'm never going to get a vacation, I won't. Have you noticed how the power of belief works in your life?

The good news is that once I changed my belief that I had to be a victim, life itself changed. And as life changed, it went right around in a circle and supported my new beliefs. Honest! All you need is a willingness to turn in your victim's role and start to look for choices. Yes, choices! Every situation in life has at least two choices. Some have more.

Thank the Experience

Sometimes it's difficult to see the choices in a situation, particularly if it's painful. I want to pass on to you something that a close friend, Virginia Miller, told me. She said that whenever you are in a situation that you don't like or don't want to be in, *thank it!* Thank the experience!

Sounds a little bizarre, doesn't it? But here's an example of what I mean. I was in a relationship with an alcoholic. It was very painful. This man was determined not to quit drinking. I was in the beginning stages of recovery from drinking and was a little shaky myself. Ginny said to me, "Echo, you've got to thank God for this experience." She said to thank the experience a hundred times a day, if that's what it would take for my pain to begin to ease. She said that even if my heart wasn't in it, I should thank God for the experience.

After a few days of half-heartedly doing this, my attitude started to change. I was seeing the experience in a different way. For instance, I started to see clearly how I had become lost in this man's alcoholism. I had lost myself because I totally focused on him. I realized I had to get back to myself and work on my own twelve-step program. I wanted to live differently. I slowly began to see how destructive the relationship was and was able to let him go. This was something that I had tried to do previously, but without success. Changing my attitude about that experience, the pain, the frustration, the powerlessness, giving thanks for the knowledge that I was learning—all these together helped me to heal that period of my life.

Many, many times over the years, when I have been in emotional pain, Ginny has lovingly reminded me to thank the experience until I feel peace inside. Can you see how doing this gets you to focus on the positive side of any situation? Simply give it a try and let yourself experience how it works.

When I was younger, my mom taught me to always look for the good in every situation. There have been many times when that's been pretty tough, but it sure is a blessing when you can do it! If we are in prison—whether literally or at our jobs, in our relationships, with our health, or with our addictions—we can set ourselves free every day with our own attitudes. We just need to be willing to see things differently.

The attitude we bring to the world each day is a twenty-four-hour-a-day choice. We can choose to be crabby, hateful, and downright nasty, or we can try to look at the whole situation in a different light. If you have the attitude that you choose your experiences in order to learn and grow, things will not be so glum. You will be excited about all of the possibilities for growth and learning. And you'll stop seeing them as static events that will never change, seeing them instead as opportunities that can reveal a new direction.

Unfortunately, most of us can't see the choices that are in each situation. For example, let's look at a work situation, where the boss or a fellow employee drives you crazy. The two of you may get into power struggles every day—a "who's right, who's wrong" sort of thing. Did it ever occur to you not to get into it in the first place? You don't have to fix blame one way or the other. You can walk away and bless the person or situation. I know that this may be the last thing you want to do, but try it anyway. When confronted with such lessons, just ask yourself this single question, "Would I rather be right or be at peace?" The results can be amazing!

If changing your attitude and blessing the situation doesn't help, then it is time to come up with another choice. Don't tell me that you have no choice. Life never gives us only one choice. I know there are some situations that seem incredibly bleak, as if there is no other choice, but life is too creative to offer us only one choice! And if life doesn't appear to offer a choice, create one for yourself. This goes back to being willing to let go of being a victim. Yes, as helpless children we are thrown into many situations in which we have no choices. We are at the mercy of others.

As adults, we can use our creative energy to come up with choices and solutions that as children we simply couldn't even imagine.

If you have something going on in your life and can't find a different solution or choice, let me give you a couple of suggestions: (1) Write down the dilemma and look at it as objectively as possible. Think of it as your best friend's problem, not yours. See what choices you could come up with then. (2) Write down your problem. Hand it to your best friend. Ask what choices she sees as solutions.

Being a victim or feeling like one is like going through life in a straitjacket. Your arms are tied, so you have no way of protecting yourself. You're dependent on other people to bail you out when you get into trouble. It's a terrible way to live! This is your life and you have every right to experience all of the goodness that life has to offer! You are the only one who can prevent this with your attitudes, beliefs, limitations, fears, self-doubt, anger, or hatred. You can stay stuck forever, or you can start asking, "Is there another way to do this?"

That's when the journey really begins!

Affirmations

Affirmations are positive statements that can help to change the way we view ourselves or the world around us. Most people, upon discovering that they are holding on to negative beliefs, try to change these by saying affirmations several times a day. For example:

Negative Belief	Affirmation
I am fat.	I am thin.
I don't deserve love.	I deserve love.
I am afraid of snakes.	I like snakes.

Through the use of repetition, affirmations can create a pattern of positive thinking in the mind. But affirmations only succeed when used in conjunction with inner work.

Messages of years past are very important to be aware of. If we are affirming what we want, but we have these messages and beliefs from the past, the results can be very mixed.

In order to change existing thinking, it's important first to understand what those beliefs really are!

For example, if you are overweight and have a belief that says, "You will always be fat because it is hereditary," all of your affirmations that "I am thin" aren't going to change that belief! The belief and the affirmation will wrestle with each other over which is going to come out on top. Or, if you feel overweight, but every day you repeat the affirmation "I am thin," your body is just going to feel confused. How can it trust such a statement when it knows it's not true . . . it really isn't thin! Similarly, if you are in financial trouble and are saying affirmations that "I am prosperous," there is going to be a huge credibility gap that your body and mind are going to pick up on. The same goes for affirmations like "I am beautiful" or "I am healthy" when they are obviously not true at the present moment.

For affirmations to work well, we have to acknowledge what is true right now and allow that truth to be reflected in the positive statement. Thus, you might also say, "I am now in the process of becoming prosperous," or "I am in the process of feeling and being attractive," or "I am in the process of becoming healthy."

If you have been saying affirmations but not getting the results you desire, you may have to go deeper in order to uncover beliefs that are getting in the way. Your body can't be tricked! Or, if you have been using affirmations, but fail to do so often or on a regular basis, you may have to step it up! Affirmations are very helpful whenever you are trying to change something in your life. But you need to say your affirmations every day, twenty to thirty times a day. Some people say them in the morning, at noon, and at night before they go to sleep.

Remember to do your part. You can't expect change to occur if you just say your affirmations each day but continue to act in the same old way. You've got to implement the necessary changes to bring about positive results. Examples of the wrong way to do this would be the person who munches on a Dove Bar while repeating affirmations that she is losing weight, or who purposely puts herself deeper in debt while affirming that she is becoming prosperous.

Along with making positive affirmations, take whatever action you must to bring the new reality into being. If you want to lose weight, eat less. If you want to be more prosperous, look for more money-making opportunities or look for ways of expanding your present business or profession. As your thinking changes, you will find yourself automatically doing more and more to ensure the outcome you desire.

If things don't begin to change after three weeks or so, the chances are that you are holding on to a negative belief that is preventing you from moving forward. For example, you might find that your body doesn't want to be thinner because putting on weight was once its way of protecting itself from physical or sexual abuse. If you are not prospering, you might be holding on to a belief that you shouldn't be wealthy because then you would have to be more responsible for your own life. If you continue to feel unattractive, perhaps it may be because your present way of being allows you to be invisible, providing a sort of camouflage so others won't notice you.

You will find that positive affirmations, joined with actions that support them, become most effective the moment you are able to rid yourself of your negative belief system. Use your journal work, particularly the work at the end of chapter 5, to support your efforts. For best results, combine your daily use of affirmations with some or all of the solutions recommended in this chapter.

Solution 9: Intuition

Deep within each one of us is a calming, soft, silent voice that speaks to us throughout the day, giving us accurate advice, direction, and guidance. We aren't meant to guess our way through life. I believe God speaks directly to each one of us through our intuition.

For as long as I can remember, my mother always referred to her intuition as her "intu." She was always saying that her "intu" told her to do this or that. My siblings and I would give her such a bad time about her "intu," but, ironically, it was always accurate. As we grew older, she encouraged each of us to listen to our own intuition. An inner knowingness, she called it.

For me, it took lots of practice to follow my mother's advice. My intellect was always fighting to be in control. I wanted to analyze my inner nudgings. It wasn't until I took a class at Unity Church, in Minneapolis, based on the book *Lessons in Truth* by Dr. H. Emilie Cady, that I realized I was doing it all backward. Cady says, "Intuition and intellect are meant to travel together, intuition always holding the reins to guide the intellect."

This seemed like an odd idea to me. I hadn't given my intuition that much credit before. When I did listen to it, its guidance was accurate. But I still did not give it much power. When I read in Cady's book, "Intuition is the open end, within one's own being, of the invisible channel ever connecting each individual with God," I changed my opinion regarding my intuition and inner voice.

That night in class, we had a wonderful discussion about intuition. It was then I realized that intuition is the inner voice of God, always directing us. I began paying much more attention to what I was feeling inside. Shakti Gawain says in her book, *Living in the Light:*

> It is often hard to distinguish the "voice" of our intuition from the many other voices that speak to us from within: the voice of our conscience, voices of our old programming and beliefs, other people's opinions, fears and doubts, rational head trips, and "good ideas."

As she suggests, I began "checking in" regularly to hear what my intuition was saying to me. I would ask God a question and then wait for the inner answer. Every time I asked for an answer, something would come, even if the inner voice was telling me to wait, be patient.

At first, I had a hard time giving up the control of my life to this inner voice. My intellect kept taking over, making all the decisions and coming up with the ideas. I went back and forth for years between letting my intellect run the show and letting God or the Universe guide me, speaking to me through my intuition.

Intuition and Health

I believe that in order for us to be and stay healthy, we need to trust and follow our intuition. Gawain writes in *Living in the Light:*

If you are willing to allow the Universe to move through you by trusting and following your intuition, you will increase your sense of aliveness and your body will reflect this with increasing health, beauty, and vitality. Every time you don't trust yourself and don't follow your inner truth, you decrease your aliveness and your body will reflect this with a loss of vitality, numbness, pain, and eventually physical disease. Disease is a message from our bodies, telling us that somewhere we are not following our true energy or supporting our feelings. The body gives us many such signals, starting with relatively subtle feelings of tiredness and discomfort. If we don't pay attention to these cues and make the appropriate changes our bodies will give us stronger messages including aches, pains, and minor illnesses. If we still don't change, a serious or fatal illness or accident may eventually occur.

If you are physically sick, you need to quiet yourself and go to that still, small voice within for guidance. You do not need to feel as if you are at the mercy of the healthcare professionals, even if they are people you have carefully chosen and have come to trust. Whenever you are required to make a decision about your healthcare, make sure you understand the available choices. Then go off by yourself and ask for guidance. It is difficult to do this when faced with a serious health challenge, but the eventual outcome is worth it. You will be saved much unnecessary pain and expense. *You will be shown what you need to do.*

Trusting Your Inner Voice

When we're not listening to and trusting our intuition, it feels like we're trying to swim upstream against the tide. It is an inner feeling of resistance that can be very wearing on our energy. When we are flowing with our inner knowingness, we feel totally alive. Now, daily, I ask God for direction or guidance in all matters. I check in with my intuition several times throughout the day. I am never disappointed. On that rare occasion, when my intellect wins out, I am always disappointed in myself for not trusting that inner voice. I have learned that it is always accurate. Always!

I have learned that there is a flow that moves through the Universe. When you tap into it, you are able to ride it like a surfer rides a wave. Suddenly, you feel a sense of oneness with the whole. It's an inner feeling of knowingness. Using it will change your life.

If you aren't sure what your intuition is or how to communicate with it, I suggest you get a copy of my book *A Still Small Voice* and read it a few times until you really get the concept of your inner voice.

Solution 10: Emotional Release

Crying is an important part of anyone's healing process. It's a way that nature gave us to release our fears, our hurts, our frustrations, and our pain, whether physical or emotional. It's one of the best ways to cleanse ourselves. Yet, so many of us see crying as a sign of weakness or are embarrassed by our tears. We fear losing control or feeling vulnerable.

Many people pride themselves on not being able to cry. I have heard clients proudly say, "I can't cry. I haven't cried in years. I don't remember the last time that I cried. You'll never see me cry. I'll never give so and so the satisfaction of seeing me cry. Crying is for babies." And then there are all the old prohibitions against boys and men crying: "Big boys don't cry. Grown men don't cry."

Let me pass something on to you that I learned at the Lifeworks clinic about vulnerability. Most people try to stay in control of their emotions, feelings, thoughts, and expressions so they won't be vulnerable. Actually, it is just the opposite. When we are flowing with life, being spontaneous, expressing our feelings, we are being vulnerable. This actually puts us in control. People who are in control in the sense of sitting on their vulnerability are actually out of control.

The scary part of giving up control is that it means we need to allow ourselves to express our feelings, our needs, our desires, our thoughts. We need to let go and learn to be spontaneous in our everyday lives, and that means if we need to cry, we need to cry *now*.

How do you feel about crying? Do you allow yourself to cry when you feel like it? Do you hold back your tears? Are you afraid of your tears? Your sadness? Your hurt feelings? Do you worry about losing control or being too vulnerable?

I used to be afraid of crying. I felt that if I really let the tears out, I would never stop. I worried that I would lose control. When I got into recovery, my sponsor encouraged me to work on crying. At first, I was so blocked that I actually had to pray and ask my Higher Power to help me release the blocks. I went to sad movies and played sad songs. But once I started crying, it seemed to come quite easily.

If you are one of those people who won't let yourself cry, I want you to ask yourself why. Don't let yourself get by with an "I don't know." Whatever block you've got about crying, you've got to get past it. The block has to be released so you can get on with this important part of your cleansing process.

If you can't figure out what your blocks to crying are, maybe you should look at how your family members expressed their sadness or hurt. If it's your pride that is keeping you from crying, consider the merits of that kind of pride!

Once you have given these questions some thought, write down in your journal whatever messages you are carrying around about crying. If you are one of those people who can't or won't let yourself cry, this exercise can be particularly important.

Finally, ask the Universe to help you cry. The answer may come in dreams, or through a friend, or in an article you read on the Internet. The Universe has a million ways of helping you overcome your blocks.

So go ahead and cry. What have you got to lose? Just lots of old, mothballed stuff that's sitting inside of your body! And who needs that?

A Note about Suicide

I'm including suicide in this section, not because I believe it to *be* a solution but because some of you may be *considering* it as a solution! Let me share with you my own experience with this important issue.

Two weeks before I quit drinking and joined a recovery program, I sat down with a full bottle of Valium and a glass of water. I was tired of the ups and downs, of hopelessness and despair. Alcohol was no longer giving me the lift that I needed. The prescription drugs I was taking seemed to keep me coasting in neutral. But it seemed impossible for me to feel good about life. I just wanted to be free from pain.

I sat on my bed, determined to kill myself. As I contemplated doing this, I had a psychic vision of Limbo. I saw many souls there, grieving the loss of their lives, wanting another chance. They were full of despair and hopelessness. A voice told me that this was where I would be going. I was so angry; I didn't want the reality of suicide slapping me in the face like that. I wanted relief, answers, solutions!

I have seen this place called Limbo in many psychic readings when clients ask about a loved one who has committed suicide. Limbo is a place halfway between our earthly plane and Heaven. It's the closest thing I have ever seen, psychically, to what Hell might be like—even though there isn't any fire and brimstone in Limbo. It is full of souls who are stuck in self-pity. This is not a place God condemns us to, should we take our own life. It is our frame of mind that condemns us to Limbo.

One concern that most of my students express when I talk about Limbo is, "Do they have help there?" or, "How come no one is helping them?" They do have help. There are guardian angels to help them out of Limbo and into Heaven, but remember that there was also help for them when they were here on Earth! They chose to ignore this offer of help, and they may choose to continue to refuse it, even in Limbo.

What happens to souls in Limbo? Once they become willing to try something other than their own solutions to their problems, to let go of their strong wills, and to surrender to other solutions besides physical death, they begin to notice the higher spirits who are offering them a way to the white light of Heaven. They are willing to reach out, and as soon as they do, help is on the way.

Once we accept that suicide can't relieve our inner pain, we become open to other solutions. That's when our healing process begins. *Whether you are here in your physical body or on the other side without your physical body, you will still need to address that inner pain.*

People get angry when I tell them about Limbo, because for so many people the prospect of suicide seems like a real option for pain relief. But clearly, this is not so! One way or another, we still have to face our inner pain and do whatever is necessary to heal it.

For those of you who have a loved one who has committed suicide, there is something you can do for that soul. Visualize him and tell him to look for the help that is available to him. Tell him to look for the white light of Heaven and go toward it. Tell him he does not need to stay stuck where he is. Say it once or twice a day. Yes, you can say it out loud. He can hear you. After a while, you will sense a release, and this is an indication that he has moved on. The sense of release is very slight, so don't get caught up in whether or not he has gone on. Simply say it until it no longer feels necessary.

Meanwhile, be assured that you can heal from whatever pain you are in. But you cannot do it by yourself. Please, if you are thinking that suicide is a solution, reach out to as many people as you can. Someone will be there to help you!

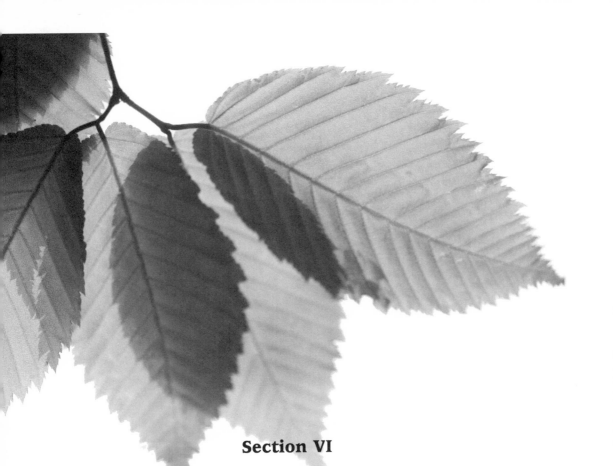

Section VI

Healing as a Way of Life

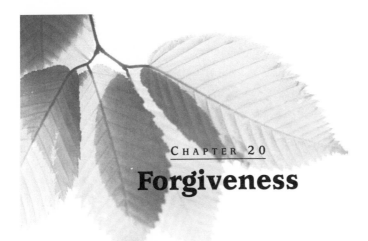

CHAPTER 20

Forgiveness

Forgiveness is a process, not an event.

As a process, it consists of stages that we move through. To begin, I would like to share these stages with you.

Stage 1:

We recognize the wrongs that have been done to us.

Forgetting is not forgiving, and denying the hurt makes it impossible for us to forgive. This stage is about remembering and then unraveling mysteries around the painful things done to us and the painful experiences we've had.

Stage 2:

We recognize that we have feelings about the wrongs.

Many of us choose to pretend that we don't have feelings

about the harm that was done to us. We take the "I don't care" or "I don't feel anything" stance. We try to blot out our feelings with food, drugs, alcohol, shopping, or gambling to distract us from the feelings of hurt, pain, anger, rage, and fear. But no matter what we do to blot them out, the fact is that we do have feelings about these hurts and it is necessary to recognize these feelings before we can at last be free of them.

Stage 3:

We embrace the feelings about the wrong.

At the Lifeworks clinics we learned how to embrace our feelings. At first, this scared me. I had spent so much of my life dodging my feelings, and now I was being told to *embrace* them. The counselor quoted M. Scott Peck, the author of *The Road Less Traveled:* "The only path away from our suffering is to embrace the suffering." Not just the physical pain, but also the emotional pain!

But what can you do if your emotional pain is stuck? If you have denied, rationalized, and minimized it for years, trying to bring it up and feel it can be very difficult. The counselor taught us to lie down on the floor in a crucifix position, arms and legs spread open, feeling completely vulnerable. He said not to do this alone, but with a couple of friends with whom you feel comfortable and safe.

Ask your body what it is holding in. Images may come; feelings may surface. Whatever comes, *go into it.* Don't resist it. This is how I got the images of all the sexual abuse that I experienced as a child. I cried, yelled, screamed, beat pillows. Whenever I would feel stuck, I'd go back into the crucifix position. Two friends held me when I needed it. They guided me through with questions. They provided a safe environment for me. It was very painful emotionally and perhaps the single most freeing experience in my life. It took less than an hour to release feelings that I had been storing for years: terror, rage, hate, fear, sadness, emptiness, abandonment, disappointment, loneliness, bitterness, and desperation.

Afterward, I was physically exhausted, but I could feel a sense of renewal in my body. My body felt free—literally unstuck. Since that day, I have done a great deal more work on embracing the liberated feelings. You can't know what this feels like until you experience the shift in your body's energy once you stop resisting and start embracing the pain. Believe me, it's wonderful!

Stage 4:

We share the feelings with others, sometimes with the wrongdoer herself.

Sharing the feelings is sharing the burden. It lessens our feelings of isolation.

Sometimes it helps to share our hurt with the person who hurt us, but in doing so you run the risk of being further abused. It is certainly not necessary. Most therapists recommend it only when a safe setting can be provided (such as with a therapist) and only under those conditions where the wrongdoer is either in recovery or is willing to work on her problems.

Our goal in this process of forgiveness is to change ourselves, not others. And the change we are seeking is a letting go of the hurt we are holding inside us. The goal of forgiveness is not to let the wrongdoer off the hook or to tell her that what she did is okay.

The goal is only to release ourselves from the pain, anger, hurt, and rage that imprison us.

Stage 5:

We make a decision about what we want to do about our relationship with the wrongdoer.

This usually evolves over time. If the wrongdoer is a family member or friend, we may need to detach from that person for a while. This can mean a period of separation from your own family if the wrongdoer is a parent, grandparent, sibling, or other close relative.

This stage may meet with resistance from other family members because it involves a change in how we operate in the system, which will have an impact on the whole family. We often feel guilty for taking care of ourselves instead of everyone else, but remember, guilt is an integral part of the family dysfunction. It is part of what we wish to heal with forgiveness. A healthy family encourages its members to do what makes them happiest and live where they want to live.

When we allow ourselves to take time away from the wrongdoer for the purpose of healing, we will heal. We will learn healthy boundaries. We will learn what kinds of relationships we want and what kinds we don't want. If and when we come back into the family, it will be under very different circumstances, and it will change the whole family dynamic. What usually happens is that you not only change the relationship between yourself and the wrongdoer, but you change the relationships of all the family members in some small or large way.

Stage 6:

There will come a sense of serenity and acceptance about the wrong and our relationships with the wrongdoer.

This is the final stage, and it does not mean that we no longer have feelings about what happened. There may always be pain or anger at the abuse or neglect. Rather, it means that the feelings we held inside us no longer control us or force us into denial. It means that our relationships no longer suffer from behavior that is inappropriate, defensive, or avoidant.

Sometimes we get stuck at one stage or another and don't complete the process. This lessens the chance for healing the relationship and reflects where we are stuck in our lives.

We also have to be prepared to reenter the forgiveness process as we receive new information or insights into how we've been hurt. Recovery itself is a lifelong process of forgiving ourselves and others. As we do this we become less and less controlled by the past.

The day finally comes when we have cleaned up all relationships from the past. This includes our relationship with ourselves. We have finished our soul's work, and are no longer stuck in blame or hatred.

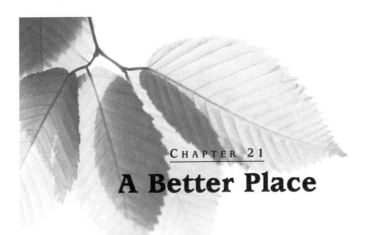

CHAPTER 21

A Better Place

Growing up with my dad was not easy. He was an alcoholic. He had a bad temper. Fortunately, he traveled for work, but when he was home, I always had a bad stomachache for fear of what was going to happen next. He was not the kind of man that should have had four kids. We made him nervous, and living with him was like walking on eggshells.

When I was fourteen he quit drinking and became a much nicer person, but he still had an edge to him that made me uneasy. Physically he was a big man—6 feet, 4 inches tall. He had been a champion boxer in the navy, and never thought twice about hitting someone. He was loud, aggressive, and demanded a lot of attention. I found out later that he had been very wounded as a child.

I could sit here and tell you story after story of some of the tough times I went through with him, but I've moved beyond those painful times to a place I like much better.

It's a place of gratitude for all that he taught me, simply by being him.

He taught me how to be self-employed and work hard. He instilled in me wonderful values and showed me the importance of treating people ethically in my business life and my personal life.

He had no prejudice, and neither do I.

He didn't force religion down my throat, but insisted I go to church every week to get a good foundation for my life.

He loved to make people happy by giving them fun presents, and that taught me to be a giving person.

His lack of patience taught me patience. His anger about his childhood taught me compassion. His devotion to God showed me that that's how I wanted to be.

He pushed himself, which has been good for me because it taught me to push myself.

He was a proud man and from him I learned the difference between good pride and destructive pride.

He went through many tough times in his life and weathered every one of them, which in turn showed me that I have that same strength and resilience.

Inner Work

Turning negative relationships into positive ones can be incredibly healing. I firmly believe there is good in every situation that we go through, but sometimes it takes real effort on our part to recognize our blessings in disguise.

You have just written an entire journal of life experiences and the majority of them have been very painful for you. I'm going to ask you to do one final piece of journaling, and that is to go back over the list of people and situations that caused you pain and find one good thing that came out of each of those experiences.

Maybe it made you a stronger person.

You learned compassion for others who have gone through it.

You stopped being a victim and took charge of your life.

Your heart was deeply wounded, but you didn't break.

You discovered that you aren't as fragile as you might have thought you were and that you're a survivor.

Yes, you were forced to grow up fast, but every situation has some gem in it. Now that you've gone through your healing process of first talking it through and then physically releasing it from your body, you should be able to see the gem.

When you see things from this new perspective, the hatred and anger seem to melt away.

Exercise 1

Hunting for Gems

Now I want you to use your journal to record the one good thing that came out of every one of the difficult experiences you've had.

Write each situation on the left side of your paper and the "Gem" on the right side of the paper. This can actually be a fun project once you get started.

Exercise 2

Giving Thanks

You can take it one step further by sending the person or people a thank-you note for all the good that came out of each experience.

Keep it focused on the good and thank each of them for the gift they gave you of finding yourself.

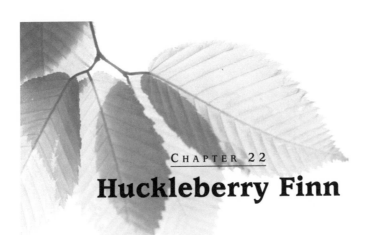

CHAPTER 22

Huckleberry Finn

W*ork consists of whatever a body is obliged to do . . . Play consists of whatever a body is not obliged to do.*

—Mark Twain

I was thinking that I had completed this book, but something just didn't feel quite finished. I could not figure out what area I had forgotten to write about. So I put a crayon in my nondominant hand and asked my inner child what area was missing. It wrote HUCKLEBERRY FINN. "What?" I asked. I could not figure out what that meant, so I asked it to tell me. It wrote FUN in big letters! "Oh," I said, "you want me to write a chapter on fun?" It replied, FUN THINGS TO DO. I thought about this. It sure felt like the missing piece. Being a person who, for a long time, hasn't been comfortable having fun, I asked others what they do for fun. See the following list of suggestions for you to think about, just in case you sometimes get stuck not knowing what to do for fun.

go to an amusement park

watch TV

read

hang out with friends

rent a movie

make a movie

go roller-skating

go for a drive

take pictures

go shopping

sew

go to the zoo

go to sporting events

play tennis

plan a party

join a club

wash your car

make T-shirts

work out at a health club

hot tub

ride your bike

go dancing

go boating

go motorcycling

go fishing

go ice skating

go bowling

do yard work

go skiing

take dance lessons

grocery shop

get a massage

fly a kite

go out to dinner

make jewelry

eat ice cream

get a new hairdo

draw pictures

go roller-blading

go to the movies

cook/bake

go swimming

play board games

go jogging

go for a walk

see a play in a theater

make a model

collect things

do volunteer work

do jigsaw puzzles

grow a garden

play an instrument

go on vacation

go to a concert

go to the races

go camping

clean your house

buy silly cards for friends

get a manicure or pedicure

mow the lawn

swing on a swing

slide down a slide

cross-country skiing

downhill skiing

sports

write poetry

gourmet cooking
go on a picnic
go hunting
knit
crochet
go hang gliding
arrange flowers
go to a museum
embroider
buy yourself a toy that you
    always wanted

go to the lake
go out to eat
go horseback riding
visit shut-ins
throw a party/entertain
pick apples
go to art festivals
go for a plane ride
collect stamps
meditate

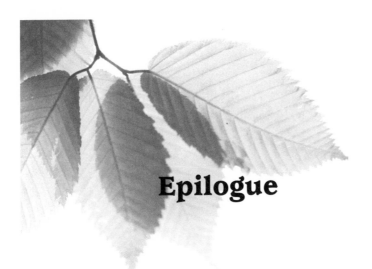

Epilogue

Here we are at the end. We've certainly traveled down a long road together.

Besides feeling sad about saying goodbye, I also feel excited for you! Once you get rid of all that old garbage, you are finally going to find out how amazing you are. You're breaking old patterns. You're no longer going to be the victim. Your life will no longer be filled with pain and self-doubt. You're taking control of your life and your destiny *and* you "deserve" every ounce of happiness that you will experience!

Carlos, a wonderful psychic friend, used to tell me to turn my scars to stars. I believe that's what I have done and that's what you're in the process of doing. By removing the pain from your memories, by healing those negative beliefs about yourself, and by looking for the good in the pain that you've endured, you, too, are turning your scars into stars.

I wish you the very best life has to offer you on your journey!

Echo

About the Author

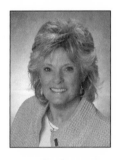

Echo Bodine first discovered her psychic abilities and the gift of healing at the age of seventeen. She enhanced her gifts with two years of training from Minneapolis-based psychic Birdie Torgeson and practiced on friends and family for twelve years before becoming a fulltime psychic, healer, and ghostbuster in 1979.

She has appeared on numerous national television shows including *Sally Jesse Raphael, Sightings, Beyond with James Van Praagh,* NBC's *The Other Side, Unexplained Mysteries,* NBC's *Today Show,* A&E, and *Encounters,* and *Paranormal Borderline* did a feature story on her family, calling them the "world's most psychic family." For two years, Echo also hosted her own cable TV show called *New Age Perspectives.*

Echo teaches psychic development at her center in Minneapolis, Minnesota, and lectures around the country on psychic abilities, spiritual healing, intuition, and ghosts. She has been writing since 1982. Her first book was *Hands That Heal,* and more recently she released *Look for the Good and You'll Find God.* This is Echo's tenth book.

Hampton Roads Publishing Company

. . . for the evolving human spirit

HAMPTON ROADS PUBLISHING COMPANY publishes books
on a variety of subjects, including spirituality,
health, and other related topics.

For a copy of our latest trade catalog, call toll-free,
800-766-8009, or send your name and address to:

HAMPTON ROADS PUBLISHING COMPANY, INC.
1125 STONEY RIDGE ROAD • CHARLOTTESVILLE, VA 22902
e-mail: hrpc@hrpub.com • www.hrpub.com